My Fight With Hospice

A Family Caring for Mom

Witness to the Misuse of Prescription Drugs

By

Andrew Weitzen

Bronze Inc.
Gainesville, FL

First Edition, April 2023
www.MyFightWithHospice.com

Library of Congress Control Number: 2023932864
ISBN: 978-1-958601-08-2 paperback
ISBN: 978-1-958601-05-1 hardcover
ISBN: 978-1-958601-09-9 ebook

Also
ISBN: 978-1-958601-10-5 audio
ISBN: 978-1-958601-03-7 hardcover Amazon no dust jacket
ISBN: 978-1-958601-02-9 paperback Amazon

Cover design by Andrew Weitzen
Cover needlepoint background by Edith Weitzen

Published by Bronze Inc.
www.Bronz.com

About This Book

I wrote this short, easy-to-read book because I was dismayed by systemic problems in medical care. This is an eyewitness account. If someone puts these institutions on trial, this is a testimony.

> I just finished reading your book. Your book is a brilliant case study. (I am qualified to make that statement. I have an MPH in epidemiology from UC Berkeley.) You have meticulously described on a definite schedule your mother's symptoms after taking specific drugs; you have also shown that these symptoms were not connected to the original cancer diagnosis. Your conclusions that her death and her suffering were both from those drugs, not cancer, is convincing (and horrifying). The problem here is that when people get a dire diagnosis for an elderly relative it is a sudden, unexpected experience and it takes a while for it to register, but they want to do something to help that relative immediately. And hospice seems the obvious solution.
>
> ~ Ann Cassin

Books by Andrew Weitzen

How To Dance With a Partner: The Gentle Method of Unambiguously Communicating Every Step in Every Social Dance invented by Andrew Weitzen - The solution to a 1,000-year-old problem. The most important advance since men and women began dancing together. www.PartnerDancing.com

My Fight With Hospice: A Family Caring for Mom, Witness to the Misuse of Prescription Drugs by Andrew Weitzen - A cautionary tale for anyone caring for family members. "Unique, touching, reflective, homage," Philip Schwartz. www.MyFightWithHospice.com

Dedication

This book is dedicated to those who have suffered from the misuse of prescription drugs; to those that have provided care for one in need; to my sisters and brother-in-law, Janet Brownstein, Randi Faris, and Stephen Brownstein for their devoted care of my mother; and to the memory of my parents Sheldon Melvyn Weitzen and Edith Berman Weitzen.

Acknowledgements

There is a Jewish tradition that the bible names people as a way of honoring them. I have tried to do the same in this book.

Author's Note

This is my story. The statements in this book are my opinions. They are not intended to represent objective facts. I do not qualify my statements by writing "in my opinion" beforehand. There may be inaccuracies, especially in the historic references to my ancestors. I did not research the past. I only related stories as told to me. Attributed quotes are how I remember them, or possibly how I wish they were said, and are not confirmed by those attributed.

I started writing this book during my mother's illness. My original title was "How I Saved My Mother from Hospice". That was not to be. I changed the title to "Why I Hate Hospice". At the end of each chapter, I had a section headed "Why I Hate Hospice" followed by a list of points. My parents had a natural empathy for others they passed on to me. I am lucky. So far, I have not felt animosity towards others regardless of how much I dislike their behavior. I do not want others to feel bad. Not being a hater, I changed the title yet again to "My Fight With Hospice" and the heading at the end of each chapter to "Issues". While I oppose the behavior of Hospice described in this book, I do not feel badly towards them. What makes me feel bad is what happened to my mother.

The Hebrew is in the public domain. The translations are my own or from the public domain, with assistance from Yosef Chodin. Any translations matching those in a copyrighted work are unintended. For the most part, I have used Hebrew from the Jewish prayer book, Siddur Ashkenaz. While I have attributed much Hebrew to Jewish prayers, the original source is often elsewhere, such as in biblical writings. The Amidah is the standing, silent meditation at the center of the Jewish service. I used Hashem, which means "The Name", for the 4 letter name of God, instead of the often used Lord.

For easier reading, I have taken some literary license in presenting the story. I have not made up any events. The quoted dialogue is as I remember. I have not made up any dialogue. As to the drugs given to my mother, this is a reasonably accurate portrayal. We wrote down every drug we gave her, along with other notes. I did not use that record for reference in this work. I wrote this story from memory. The technical information about drugs I got from various websites. Where I have consolidated information into my own words, I have not attributed references. The same information is widely available in the public domain. You can do your own research. My purpose here is to question, not to convince.

I knew next to nothing when my mother was diagnosed. I had no specific agenda against Hospice, the medical field, or the drug industry. Unlike many others, I was not somebody who said, "I am going to research everything on cancer to save my mother." I assumed she would get properly treated according to her wishes. Only after I was shocked at the medical treatment my mother received did I begin to investigate. I stayed in the room with my mother most days and nights for four and a half months. I spent countless hours reading about cancer, drugs, and nutrition during my mother's illness.

My mother's end was horrible. I have deliberately left off descriptions of my mother's suffering. I have included enough for you to know how she suffered so you could feel sympathetic. I avoided going into details to keep you from sharing her suffering, so you would not feel empathetic. I am seeking your understanding, not your commiseration. The horror my mother suffered was caused by Hospice. Hospice saw the same events differently. They blamed my mother's suffering on cancer. They accepted turning my mother into a drug addict as natural. They refused to acknowledge the drugs as the cause of my mother's suffering.

My sisters and brother-in-law could not have provided more devoted care for my mother. No person could have received more attention than my mother did as one of us was always with her. However, my sisters believed Hospice instead of me. I was fighting against four people, my mother, my two sisters, and my brother-in-law, in my battle to save my mother from Hospice. For the most part, I have left out the role my sisters played in my mother's care. When I write "we" as in "we took my mother", I mean myself and one or more of my family members. When I write Mom choose something or Hospice did something, I mean with the support of my sisters.

I believe Hospice put my mother through months of unnecessary suffering. I believe Hospice deprived my mother, us, family, and friends of having meaningful experiences. I joked Hospice kept my mother from enjoying her cancer. As I write this two months after her passing, I believe my mother would still be alive if Hospice had not killed her. Perhaps I should say euthanized her because this seems like what they do.

Hospice could not have done what they did without the support of my sisters. My sister had power of attorney over my mom's healthcare. If I would have had the power of attorney, Mom would not have been under Hospice care. I love my sisters and they loved our mother. I do not blame them. I consider my sisters victims. They were not my mother's doctors. They did not prescribe the drugs. They believed the "professionals", as my sister called the Hospice workers. I write this account so you will not be so naive. You will form your own opinion. When your time comes, if you read this, you will not be caught so unaware. Maybe you can save a loved one.

Take Action

Since writing this book, many people have come forward with similar stories. People are angry about what happened. They want something done. The first step in affecting change is awareness.

Send Your Story and This Book

The most effective way to bring about change is to go directly to those with the power to make a difference. Send your story along with this book to your healthcare providers, hospice, and government representatives. Let them know of your concerns. Their job is to protect the public welfare. Most of them want to do the best they can. They need your help. Keep them informed.

Celebrities

Prescription drugs are the third leading cause of death in the United States and Europe. Half die that have taken their drugs correctly. Half die because of errors such as too high a dose or use of a drug despite contraindications. ~ Pol Arch Med Wewn. 2014;124(11): PMID: 25355584.

Some celebrity victims of prescription drugs.

Louisa May Alcott
Lenny Bruce
Kurt Cobain
Truman Capote
Dorothy Dandridge
Tommy Dorsey
Brian Epstein
Sigmund Freud
Judy Garland
Jimi Hendrix
Abbie Hoffman
Howard Hughes
Philip Seymour Hoffman

Whitney Houston
Michael Jackson
Alan Ladd
Heath Ledger
Bruce Lee
Margaux Hemingway
Marilyn Monroe
Brittany Murphy
Prince Rogers Nelson
Tom Petty
Elvis Presley
Joan Rivers
Anna Nicole Smith

Contents

Prologue: A Rat on the Bird Feeder

בָּרוּךְ אַתָּה ה' אֱלֹהֵינוּ מֶלֶךְ הָעוֹלָם. פּוֹקֵחַ עִוְרִין.

Blessed are You Hashem our God, King of the
Universe, Who allows the blind to see.

~ Jewish morning blessing upon opening your
eyes

"There is a rat on the bird feeder," shrieked my mother in
revulsion.

I came running.

The bird feeder was squirrel-proof. A spring attached to
the perch opened a window for the birds to get the seeds. The
squirrels were too heavy for the spring. When the squirrels
climbed on the perch, the window closed.

The rat was smarter than the squirrels. The rat figured
out that when he jumped up from the perch the window
opened briefly enough for him to dart his paw in to grab some
seeds.

My mother could not get rid of that bird feeder fast
enough. She gave the bird feeder to my sister.

Part I Winning the First Battle With Cancer

בָּרוּךְ אַתָּה ה' אֱלֹהֵינוּ מֶלֶךְ הָעוֹלָם אֲשֶׁר יָצַר אֶת הָאָדָם
בְּחָכְמָה וּבָרָא בוֹ נְקָבִים נְקָבִים חֲלוּלִים חֲלוּלִים. גָּלוּי וְיָדוּעַ
לִפְנֵי כִסֵּא כְבוֹדֶךָ שֶׁאִם יִפָּתֵחַ אֶחָד מֵהֶם אוֹ יִסָּתֵם אֶחָד
מֵהֶם אִי אֶפְשַׁר לְהִתְקַיֵּם וְלַעֲמוֹד לְפָנֶיךָ אֲפִילוּ שָׁעָה אֶחָר .

Blessed are You Hashem Our God, King of the universe, Who had formed human beings in wisdom and created within them many hollow openings. ... If one opening was closed or if one was opened, a person could not survive for even a short time.

~ Asher Yatzor, That was Formed, Jewish blessing after going to the bathroom

Chapter 1 Edie

You are our flesh and blood. We love you no matter what.

~ Edith Weitzen

When I was in college, I told my mother I did not know what I wanted to do with my life. My mother said, "I am 45 years old and I still do not know what I want to do with my life."

My mother passed away on Sunday, July 17, 2016, at 5:18 pm. She was 84 years old. Looking at that number now seems old, but only a year before Mom seemed healthy with many active years to come. She had healthy friends that were 90, that were not in as good shape as her at her age. Mom's last moments were peaceful. My sister Janet and I were with her, holding her hands. We said the Shema for her, which Jews traditionally say with their last breath. In English the words are "Hear O Israel, the Lord our God, the Lord is One." We put pants on her since she only had on a diaper and a shirt.

We are lucky. Judaism has prescribed customs for dealing with death. There is little for us to figure out. We called the Rabbi, Hospice, and the funeral home. Rabbi Kaiman came over and read a blessing. Hospice came over, took down the death information, and gathered up the drugs. The funeral home people took Mom away. Janet did not want to watch, but I watched. Watching was tough. The Rabbi notified whomever he needed to. We called family and friends. The process was in motion.

In Judaism, life is for the living. We bury our dead as soon as possible. The Chevra Kadisha, holy friends, washed Mom's body and put her body in a shroud. Someone stayed with her body until the funeral. Relatives flew into town on Monday.

Tuesday morning, at 10:30 am, only 42 hours after Mom passed away, we were at the synagogue for the ceremony.

Our funeral ceremonies are short. Janet spoke for a few minutes. She is a good writer and funny. She stole some of my material that I had written for the obituary. I spoke next. I said, "I wrote some of that." I told everyone Janet was worried we were going to overlap. I said we were a little. Janet wanted to talk about her relationship with Mom. I wanted to give them a feeling of what Mom was like. Here is what I said.

Mom lived a great life, a long life. She spent 50 years with her first choice, my dad, and her best friend. They raised three healthy children. They loved their life.

Every part of Mom's life she made dear friends whom she loved and who loved her.

After my dad passed away, Mom was feeling sorry for herself and said, "Nobody wants to do anything with me."

I told her that she was not on people's schedules right now. She was like the new kid on the block, but that would change. She would get on people's schedules. Others would join her situation. She would not be the new person anymore.

Over the last ten years, she embraced and was embraced by a wonderful group of ladies and men, the lunch bunch, the knitting circle, the book club, the opera group, and her longtime friends, to have a lovely, meaningful life after my dad's passing. What a beautiful community we have here.

I want to tell you how much all of you have meant to my mother, Janet, Randi, and me, throughout all the years and for the last few months for all the calls, letters, gifts, and support.

My mother, was born Edith Berman on April 17, 1932, to Ida Bossman and Philip Berman. She grew up with her beloved, older brother Sol on Coney Island surrounded by her Jewish, Russian immigrant family in a house with grandparents, uncles, and relatives. For her first five years, her native language was Yiddish. They were from the old country. They were observant. They washed the floors before Shabbos with newspapers. My mother was a sophisticated young woman. She did not appreciate the old ways.

One day her grandmother said to her, "I am going to die now,". Her grandmother laid down in my mother's bed and passed away. My mother thought she saw her grandmother's spirit fly around the room before leaving.

Mom was a child of the beach and parks. She was athletic, she swam, she played tennis, and she played ping pong. Her mother walked miles every day. Mom did the same. For the last decade, Sandy Shuster was Mom's walking buddy.

Yes, Mom could dance. My parents did the Lindy. No, she did not show me how. She did not know the steps. She just did them. If you want to learn the Lindy, come out on Monday nights to my dance class.

Mom loved to laugh and make people laugh. She had a street full of childhood friends she kept her whole life. They were a lively crowd, each trying to outdo the other. My dad was the same way.

They were from depression era, Jewish immigrant families. They lived through World War II. They were right out of the movies, from the same neighborhood as Mel Brooks, Neil Simon, and Woody Allen. They laughed, they yelled, they fought. They were living life, like the old joke, two Jews having a discussion sound like four Americans having an argument. In New York, my parents were one of the bunch, but in Florida people were not used to that, and my parents were the life of the party.

Mom was a natural beauty inside and out. After high school her friends got married. Mom went to Brooklyn College on scholarship. While walking around campus, a pageant organizer asked her to be in the most beautiful girl on campus contest. Janet's friends called her Edie with the hot body. When I was in high school, she thought she embarrassed me by wearing a white bikini. Maybe she did. My parents thought that was funny.

My cousin Ruth loved my parents. She said, "Your mother was so beautiful, and she was kind." Yes, she was. After my dad's factory closed my dad had a cleaning business. Grady Bridges, the main guy that worked for my dad, got evicted from his home. My mom and dad went over. Mom said it "was the saddest thing you ever want to see. All their stuff taken out of their house and them standing in the street." My parents helped gather up their stuff and found them a place to live.

Mom made others feel good to be around her. She was a great listener. Some friends that had moved away were having trouble. One day the husband called my mother. I heard my mother tell him, "I do not know what is wrong with her. She is crazy." Soon after, the wife called. My mother told her, "You have to do what you have to do." She understood what people were feeling. They felt better having talked with her.

My Mom met my dad on her 21 birthday at a Jewish singles party. Her mother Ida was a master seamstress. My mom was wearing a body-hugging, knit red dress that her mother made for her. My dad was a big, handsome guy. They must have seen each other. My dad took her out from a crowd of guys.

The next day they had their first date. My dad said he had a friend who had a place on Fire Island. The boat my dad took out broke down. They got out of the boat and waded across the marsh. When they got to the house, the door was locked. My dad broke in. Nothing would deter him.

My mom had not met anyone like that before. She told my dad, "Every summer I have a romance, but at the end of the summer, I do not want you getting any ideas. It is good by Charlie time."

Summer ended and my mom wanted to get married.

My dad said, "But it is good by Charlie time."

She went to Texas. He wrote her a letter. We have the letter. The letter is not very good. She came back.

My dad still would not take my mom out on Saturday nights, because that was too serious.

Mom was determined to get married and had another guy. One day my dad was over at my mom's and the other guy drove up. My mom pushed my dad into the bushes. As she talked to the other guy, my dad thought, "This is not good, me hiding in the bushes."

They got married. My dad told me, "I got lucky."

Mom was a soul full of life. I tried to give you a little of that feeling.

Before I moved back to Gainesville, I was up here visiting. I saw how Mom and Dad watched my nephew Josh during the day. First Mom had Josh. She spent the morning with him. She gave him her attention the entire time. She played games with him, but not kids' games, they were reading games. She was educating him.

When she was done, my dad had Josh for the afternoon. My dad and Josh had built a model town with a parking lot. Josh and Dad were in business parking cars. They learned the names of all the cars then went into the office, added up the receipts, and took the profits to go buy ice cream.

I have never seen anything like that, the attention my nephew got from my parents every day. Well, maybe I have. My parents loved being parents. Watching them with Josh was like a time machine into my childhood.

My mom had a cool Uncle Harry who had a stereo optic camera. My dad was the executor of Harry's estate. My dad found a viewer and stereo optic photos Harry had taken at Janet's first birthday party in 1960. We have 3D images of my parents from when they were young parents. It is really something to see my mom in 3D when she was 26. I can tell you when I was taking care of her, I did not see an old lady. I saw that 26-year-old, young mother at heart.

We will be sitting Shiva this week through Sunday. You are invited to come over. There will be services at my house at 6 pm every evening, except Friday and Saturday services will be here at the synagogue. If you want to come when there are a bunch of folks, come then. If you would like to come when things are quiet, come during the days or in the evening. Monday morning, around 10, I will go for the ceremonial walk around the neighborhood to end Shiva. You are invited to join me.

Janet, Randi, and I got lucky. We had great parents. We have been lucky to have you, great family, and friends.

Chapter 2 Escitalopram

I got lucky when I married your mother.

~ Sheldon Weitzen

Escitalopram

Brand name Lexapro. Selective serotonin reuptake inhibitor (SSRI). Can treat depression and generalized anxiety disorder (GAD).

Your mental health may change in unexpected ways including these symptoms: worsening depression, thinking about harming or killing yourself, extreme worry, agitation, panic attacks, aggressive behavior, irritability, acting without thinking, severe restlessness, and frenzied abnormal excitement.

Common side effects include blurred vision, diarrhea, drowsiness, dry mouth, fever, frequent urination, headache, indigestion, nausea, influenza-like symptoms, pain in neck or shoulders, increased or decreased appetite, and weight changes.

Right after Thanksgiving in 2015, Mom had a pain in her hip. She stopped walking, felt depressed, and went to see her doctor. She said she knew she needed anti-depression medication to get better. She had gotten depressed a few times in the past when she was sexually harassed by the school principal where she was teaching, when my dad had lost his business, and when my dad passed away. She said only the medication got her out of the depression. Her doctor put her on Escitalopram, possibly another medication first. The doctor missed his chance to detect her cancer at that time, or even earlier, as she had been seeing him for years.

In the fall of 1980, I was living with my parents. I got a call from my childhood friend Peter Ritter. "What are you doing?" Peter asked.

I had graduated college in the spring and had hung around all summer waiting for a job in Georgia to come through, for which my dad had arranged. "Not much," I said, "Writing software on my dad's Apple computer."

"Come to New York. You can live with us," said Peter.

I flew to New York with my dad. He gave me a return plane ticket and an evening job in his small sales office. My day job was looking for a job. The job in my dad's office paid $5 per hour for writing software for Joe Geller. Among Joe's many duties was systems analysis. Our software was to help with pricing the shirts they manufactured. The office was in the Empire State Building. Peter lived at 31 E 31 Street, near Madison Avenue, not far from the Empire State Building. Every day on my way to and from work I peeked in the one-of-a-kind game store The Compleat Strategist.

Peter's roommate was his best friend from high school Richard Porter, the Dickster. The Dickster was an advertising executive on Madison Avenue. He used to say, "Do you know how you make a product hot? You go around telling everybody the product is hot. It is all smoke and mirrors." The Dickster went on to have a major career in advertising, becoming the publisher of Woman's Day, Readers Digest, and TV Guide, the most widely distributed magazines in the world.

Peter and Dickey lived in a converted loft the size of a one bedroom apartment with three other guys: Mike McNamara, the Mikester, Stan, and Mark Mandel. The Dickster had the best space, a curtained-off bedroom area in the back of the apartment, with his own TV. Peter had the bedroom area on the top of a low loft in the front of the apartment. Stan lived in the Hole under Peter's space. The Mikester had the high loft above the couch in the living room, which faced the group TV.

Mark was a college friend of the Dickster's. Mark was the last one in and had the least desirable space, the couch. The couch afforded no privacy. You could not go to sleep until everyone left the living room. After three months, Mark's stay was over. He had to move on. The next three months were my turn on the couch, for which I paid $25 per week.

By the end of my three months, I found a job working for Alexander and Alexander as a computer programmer in actuarial consulting at the insurance brokerage. I moved out and sublet Miriam Isaacs' apartment in nearby Murray Hill. Miriam, a salesperson for my dad, had gone back to Israel for the time being.

In the middle of winter, I told my boss New York was too cold. I was going back to Florida, or on to Texas or California. He laughed. He asked me to stay for a couple more months.

Miriam came back. I moved in with my grandmother Bertha in Brighton Beach in Brooklyn. I worked in Steven's Tower in mid-town Manhattan on the west side near Rockefeller Center. Conveniently the D train went direct from my grandmother's block to the basement of Steven's Tower. I did not have to change trains. The ride took one hour.

Grandma was depressed after Grandpa Joe had passed away. She was taking anti-depressant medication, perhaps even Escitalopram. My uncle Jerry said my moving in with Grandma did her a lot of good.

After a couple of months, my job ended. I went back to Florida, then to California to look for a new job. Had I understood more about what was going on with my grandmother, I might have stayed with her longer.

Chapter 3 Bertanini

Your Mom was special. May I share a bit of personal history with you? When I was growing up and had to deal with an insensitive stepfather your Mom often played the go-between. She somehow found a way to talk to this difficult man on my behalf. Her sense of fairness and courage has never been forgotten by me.

~ Cousin David Bossman

According to my dad's cousin Morris, the great Lefkowitz married a very beautiful woman. They lived in the Austrian Hungarian Empire in the area of the Carpathian Mountains. They had 12 children. Leah, one of those Lefkowitz children, married Mordecai Steinberg. They had eight children. The oldest was my grandmother Bertha Steinberg.

Morris said Mordecai was a great man. Mordecai was conscripted into the army, found himself in Siberia, and walked home. He was gone seven years. Mordecai had a long beard. Morris laughingly says, on Friday nights before Shabbos, Mordecai, on his way home, would stop at each of the cousins' houses for a shot of schnapps. The Nazis cut off Mordecai's beard before they killed him.

The Steinbergs had Bertha, Julie, Rudy, Bernie, Irving, Louie, Adolph, who died young in the army from a fever, and Mendel. Bertha was born at the beginning of the twentieth century. As a young woman, after the Great War, Bertha came with a friend to the United States. Bertha was fixed up with another Hungarian Jew and married him, my grandfather Joseph Weitzen. We say Hungarian, but when they did not want their kids to know what they were saying, they spoke Ukrainian.

Bertanini, as she was known to the cousins, became the matriarch of the family. Between the wars, she helped her brothers come to the United States. After World War II, she helped displaced relatives come to the United States. She put people up in her house. She found them places to live, jobs, and spouses.

In Europe, Bertha's sister Julie married Abraham Sternberger. They had four children, Morris, Laura, and two older boys, Ludwick and Alex. Morris' older brother Alex saved Morris' life in Auschwitz. During a lineup, Morris' father saw the Nazis calling names of smaller adolescents. Morris' father told Alex, "When the Nazis call Morris' name, you step out instead." When Alex stepped out, the Nazis saw how big he was and told him to step back in line. Julie did not live through the war.

At the end of the war, when the Russian army was approaching, the Nazis evacuated the Jews on what became a death march. Morris' father and older brothers did not survive the march. Morris did, losing his toes to frostbite.

Laura, Morris' sister, did survive the war. Laura and Morris, independently, made their way to the United States and were taken in by my grandmother Bertha. When Morris saw my grandmother, he cried. He thought she was his own mother. They looked so much alike. Morris and Laura both married, had children and grandchildren and now live happily in South Florida. They are 89 and 87 years old respectively. You can watch Morris' oral history video interview on the US Holocaust Memorial Museum website as part of the Shoah project.

Joe Weitzen was born in 1895. He had five sisters and a brother. The Weitzens left Europe for the Bronx before World

War I. Joe had a cousin Eddie Weitzen. When Eddie went into the army, he scored so high on the IQ test that he ended up on General Omar Bradley's staff. Joe's father was Avraham Moshe. When a male child was born in the family, Joe would say, "No one is named after my father", which is why my older cousin is named Arthur and I am Andrew Mark, our Hebrew names both being Avraham Moshe.

Joe and Bertha moved their family to Brighton Beach before my dad's bar mitzvah. On the one-year anniversary of my dad's bar mitzvah, according to the Hebrew calendar, Joe took my dad to the synagogue. My dad had not been to synagogue much and did not know this was the anniversary of his bar mitzvah. When the time came to read the haftorah, Joe bid on and won the honor. Joe turned to my dad and said, "Go read. This is the portion from your bar mitzvah." You can imagine how embarrassed my dad was, as he was unprepared to read the haftorah in Hebrew. Joe was a sweet man. He passed away at the age of 84 from lung cancer. He did not smoke much, only an occasional cigar.

When I moved in with my grandmother Bertha in 1981, she lived in the same apartment in Brighton Beach that my dad had moved into some 40-plus years earlier. This was the same apartment that so many of the relatives had lived in many years before. I was the last of the relatives to live with her. Grandma Bertha was 79 years old, strong, and in good health. When I came home from work, she cooked me dinner. She did everything on her own like she had her entire life. My dad said she could have lived to 90.

Joe had died a few years earlier. Grandma was lonely. Though she was the oldest, all her brothers had passed away. Bernie, who was a bachelor, had lived with her and Joe. Bernie's passing before Grandpa had been a shock to Grandma. She thought Bernie would outlive her and keep her company. My dad's sister, my aunt Lorraine, lived in Manhattan. She came to visit Grandma often. Sometimes the three of us would sit in the apartment. I would watch TV and exercise, while the two of them sat crying.

A few months after I moved out, the family had an 80 birthday party for Bertha. A few months after that, Bertha jumped off the roof of her apartment building. She had pinned a note to her blouse, "I am Bertha Weitzen. I live in apartment 2D. I miss Joe."

Her cousins blamed her death on the antidepressant medication. I believe them. Go back to the last chapter to read the warnings for Escitalopram.

Chapter 4 Too Late

> I miss your mother. I cannot believe she is gone.
> She was the most youthful of everyone.
>
> ~ Marian Cohen, neighbor and friend of 45+
> years

In 2005 I moved in with my mother. My father had passed away in the fall of 2003. My mother was living alone for the first time in her life. I had been living in Boca Raton, then New York and then Chicago. The job I was working on ended. Since I had no other place to be, I decided to temporarily move in with my mom to keep her company. I did not want my mother to be lonely like my grandmother.

My sister Janet lived one mile away. She had moved her family back to Gainesville several years before so my parents could help raise her children. While Janet's children were now in college, my mother still went to Janet's house daily to do various things.

One day when my mother was in her 80s, a friend Jesse said to me, "Your mother is amazing." While Jesses's mom was struggling, my mother was strong physically and mentally healthy. She walked every day, worked in the yard, went up and down the steps in our house and took care of herself completely.

At the end of February 2016, two months after going to see the doctor about being depressed, my mom went to lunch with her friends. They called themselves the lunch bunch. My mom's hip was hurting so bad that they cut their lunch short to bring my mother home.

Though they did not know, for them my mother died that day. That was the last time any of them saw or talked with my mother. See the appendix for a sample of the notes they sent my mother during my mother's illness.

The next day, we called an ambulance to take Mom to the hospital. My sister Janet, the doctor, stayed with Mom. I went home. After some tests, my sister called me. Mom had stage IV lung cancer, which metastasized to her hip.

On the front page of the newspaper that day was an article about lung cancer. That day was a special day promoting awareness about lung cancer. The article said there were new treatments that meant advanced lung cancer was no longer a death sentence. The story was about a woman, now in her 70s, who had the same diagnosis as my mother. The woman had been through chemotherapy that did not help. Her doctor put her on a new drug Tarceva®, which shrunk her tumors. This woman was still doing well after seven years. I took the article with me as I went back to the hospital.

Too late. By the time I got to my mom's hospital room, my mom had already made up her mind that she was not going to be treated. She was going to live at my sister's under the care of Hospice. She could not have made a worse decision.

There was no talking to my mom at that point. From what I understand, my mom was told she had the worst diagnosis possible, she had stage IV lung cancer, the cancer had spread throughout her body, there was no cure and she was going to die a horrible death. My mom believed she only had a week or two to live.

Mom said she wanted to take a pill that would put her to sleep so she would not wake up in the morning. I said thank god that was illegal in Florida. As things turned out, my mother was right. Due to the suffering Hospice ended up inflicting on my mother, a pill right then would have saved my mother much misery. Things did not have to turn out that way.

To get a diagnosis of no hope with the promise of a painful death is terrible. This was the first disaster in Mom's care, frightening my mom into paralysis so she would not consider treatment.

The diagnosis was not true. The cancer had not spread throughout her body. The cancer had metastasized to two places only, her hip and back, which could both be treated with radiation. The cancer in her lung was slow growing. She was not going to die the following week. There were non-aggressive treatment options.

I would have presented my mother with a much different scenario. I would have started by telling Mom there is good news and bad news. The good news is there is a woman on the front page of today's paper that has the same diagnosis, has lived for seven years and is doing well taking a pill. Many other people are doing just as well taking the same pill.

I was too late though. Mom would not listen to any of that. She was medicated by the hospital staff. She was uncharacteristically anxious. Looking back, I suspect the drugs were making her crazy. She was not in her right mind. She was unable to rationally consider her options. This was still her first day in the hospital. She had not seen her doctor yet.

To be fair to Hospice, I could have titled this book "What I Hate About the Medical System". Already, my mother was over-medicated before seeing anyone that would treat her. I think the hospital had her on Oxycodone and Lorazepam in addition to the Escitalopram. She should not have been on any of them. The pain in her hip was only when she stood up, not when sitting in bed. She certainly did not need Lorazepam to calm her down. Later on, we saw she had an adverse reaction to the Lorazepam that made her nuts. I cannot think straight if I miss out on an hour of sleep. How can anyone think straight on three mind altering drugs? I hate that my mother was robbed of her rationality.

Issues With the Hospital

1. Over-medication as a matter of practice when under-medication should be the norm.

Chapter 5 Smoke and Mirrors

She was a very dear friend and I have so many fond memories of our good times together. She was so special and the kind of friend that comes along so rarely in one's lifetime.

~ Rochelle Hester

The morning of Mom's second day in the hospital, her doctor, a gerontologist, came early to see her to give her the diagnosis. The doctor arrived to find that my mother already had the diagnosis prematurely. Later, he told me she was so stressed that she would not let him discuss seeing the oncologist and radiation oncologist which he thought she should do. Once again, I attribute my mother's irrational behavior to the drugs she was on.

While my mother did not want to see the oncologist or radiation oncologist, she was willing to see Hospice. How did my mother come to this decision to see Hospice rather than an oncologist? Hospice has a marketing message that appears to come straight from the Dickster's Madison Avenue wisdom, "How do you make a product hot? Tell everyone the product is hot."

What does Hospice tell everyone? "The important thing is to keep you comfortable." I heard this message repeated to me from multiple places, one being the synagogue. Later on, I heard this message come back to me from a surprising source. From a thousand miles away, my cousins Bill and Leah said, "The important thing is to keep her comfortable." That is how well Hospice has branded this message.

Hospice came by during the day to make their sales pitch to my mom on what they do. Hospice has expanded their service. In addition to end-of-life care, which my mother was not ready for, Hospice now offered palliative care. Hospice provides you with a hospital like bed, portable toilet and other accoutrements for your care. They also have a nurse and healthcare worker come to your house for regular visits. A social worker comes now and then. You are under the care of the Hospice doctor.

End-of-life care is for your last days during which you will have no treatment to make you better. Palliative care, according to the National Cancer Institute, is given to improve the quality of life of patients. In the appendix of this book, you can find a more complete explanation of palliative care provided by the National Cancer Institute.

My mom bought into Hospice's pitch on palliative care. She took Hospice's message of comfort at face value. She thought she would go home and Hospice would keep her comfortable. This message is false. My mother did not spend one day comfortably. Nearly all her misery was caused by Hospice's medical treatment.

Though they say they do, Hospice does not provide palliative care. Hospice only knows one type of care, end-of-life care. They treat their palliative care patients the same as they treat their end-of-life patients. Hospice does not try to make you better. Hospice does no diagnosis. Hospice administers drugs, without knowing, or wanting to know, what is wrong. Hospice does not treat you. Hospice treats symptoms to keep you quiet, not comfortable.

While you are under Hospice's care, Hospice prohibits you from getting any kind of treatment other than palliative care. This is fine for an end-of-life provider, but not for a palliative care provider. According to the National Cancer Institute, "The goal of palliative care is to prevent or treat, as early as possible, the symptoms and side effects of the disease and its treatment." "The goal is to maintain the best possible quality of life." "Often, palliative care specialists work as part of a multidisciplinary team ... [which] may consist of ... doctors, nurses, registered dieticians ... psychologists." "Palliative care is given in addition to cancer treatment."

Hospice should not be in the palliative care business. Being a palliative care provider is a conflict of objective with being an end-of-life care provider. One doctor cannot service both these roles.

My mother should not have been a candidate for Hospice. Hospice should not have accepted my mother as a patient. Hospice should have referred my mother to the oncologist. Only when you are on death's door and there are no other options should you be under Hospice's care.

How was my mother a candidate for Hospice? To be a candidate for Hospice, you must have a diagnosis to live six months or less. When I asked my mother's gerontologist how long Mom had to live, he said he did not know. He said some people pass away in a couple of weeks, others years, but most within a few months. My mother's gerontologist gave my mom a diagnosis of two weeks to six months. He did this so she would be eligible for Hospice. He did not do her any favors.

I have so many problems with this type of medical practice. This is an example of the insidiousness of the system. While I do not believe this is an outright conspiracy, the effect is the same. The gerontologist knows Hospice's rules, so he gives my mother a diagnosis based on Hospice's rules. The phrase ass-backwards comes to mind. The gerontologist is not qualified to determine how long my mother is going to live. My mother had not even had a biopsy done to determine what kind of cancer she had. He is not an expert in the field of lung cancer.

How dare anyone give someone else a diagnosis of how long the other person is going to live? No one knows the answer to this question on an individual basis. Medical care should be about treating individuals. How long someone lives is dependent on their behavior and their care. What he should have said was, if you take the best care of yourself, you eat the best foods, you get the best treatment options, we do not know how long you will live. Note the lady in the newspaper still going strong after seven years. On the other hand, if you let Hospice care for you, turn you into a drug addict, keep you bedridden, shutdown your bowels, and keep you constipated; and you eat the worst foods, you will probably suffer miserably and be dead in a few months. This is what happened.

To be fair to Hospice, at this time, Hospice was not the one who gave my mother a diagnosis of 6 months or less.

Issues With the Doctor

1. Making an unqualified diagnosis of how long Mom was going to live based on criteria for acceptance to Hospice's care.

Issues with Hospice

1. Not putting the patient's interest first.

2. Misrepresenting what they do.

3. Misrepresenting what is going to happen to you under their care.

4. Depriving my mother of making an informed decision.

Chapter 6 Oncologists

When I first met your parents, the neighborhood changed. Your mother and dad were so special and unique. ... I remember how Edie laughed when I brought crackers with my chopped liver on Passover. What humor and joy. There was always something fun going on at the Weitzen household. Your mom was an original. Your dad too!

~ Carole Birndorf

While still in the hospital, my mother agreed to see the oncologist and the radiation oncologist. This way, they could come by her hospital room without us having to take Mom to their offices. The radiation oncologist came by first. He explained about the tumors in Mom's hip and back. He told us they could do palliative radiation to treat these tumors. He said, "It would be a shame, if a year from now, you were in pain the whole time. We can treat these tumors, which will cause them to shrink and relieve the pain."

Treating these tumors was crucial. Tumors in the bone are painful. The tumor in Mom's left hip was what caused her to go to the hospital. Without treating these tumors Mom would be bedridden. That would be a disaster. If the treatment went well, Mom could be mobile and live her life. I fought with my mom. She agreed to go to the radiation oncologist the following week after she went home to my sister's house.

The oncologist also came by while Mom was still in the hospital. The oncologist told my mother that there was a pill that could shrink the tumors depending on what variation her cancer was. When the lab results from the biopsy came back, we would know if she was a candidate for that pill.

My mom did not want chemotherapy or surgery or extensive radiation. Thirty years ago my mom's best friend Barbara Goldstein died of breast cancer. Mom was with Barbara through Barbara's treatment. Mom did not want to go through the same thing. Cancer treatment today is not like treatment was thirty years ago. Treatment is more targeted. Side effects are less. Results are better.

The oncologist that visited my mother was from the same office that treated the lady in the newspaper. Their office has a superb reputation. Someone told me a story of a friend of theirs that first went to that same office. They then went to the most prestigious cancer centers in the country. After shopping around, they decided this office was the best one for them.

The oncologist can provide palliative care. You are much better off having the oncologist provide palliative care than Hospice. The oncologist runs tests to see what is wrong with you then prescribes the appropriate treatment.

Mom was medicated. She was not herself. She believed she was going home to die the next week. She wanted to get out of the hospital. She did not want to deal with her situation. My mother was terrified of the oncologist and comforted by Hospice, so Mom choose Hospice. She should have felt the other way around.

I did not want to go along with my mother's decision. When you are under emotional distress, you cannot be trusted to make the best choice for yourself. You may make choices to relieve the distress without regard for the consequences which may be worse. You need people around you whom you can trust who can help you make good decisions. You need someone looking out for you. I was determined to look out for my mom. My plan was to have her bone tumors treated with radiation to relieve her pain and give her mobility. I thought once that happened she would accept her situation, engage with her friends, and live her life.

If you get cancer, you are crazy not to see the oncologist. The oncologists train their whole life for this moment. They have countless patients like you. My mother would have been much better off under the care of the oncologist. I believe my mother would have gotten back to living her life, for however long, if she were under the oncologist's care. This was the one and only time my mother saw the oncologist.

Once my mother was a patient of Hospice, Hospice would not allow my mother to see the oncologist. As you know now, this is fine for an end-of-life provider but wrong for a palliative care provider. To see the oncologist, we would need to fire Hospice.

Issues With Hospice

1. Depriving my mother of seeing the oncologist.

Chapter 7 Oxycodone

Your parents were larger than life.

~ Barbara Oberlander

Oxycodone

Opioid pain medication, also called a narcotic. Works in the brain to change how your body feels pain.

High risk for addiction and dependence. Can slow or stop your breathing. More likely to cause breathing problems in older adults and people who are severely ill, malnourished, or otherwise debilitated.

Side effects include stomach pain, nausea, vomiting, constipation, loss of appetite, confusion, severe drowsiness, headache, lightheadedness, dizziness, and mild itching. To prevent constipation, eat a diet adequate in fiber, drink plenty of water, and exercise.

Practical recommendations for opioid prescription in the elderly include meticulous review of indication for opioid use, not only initially but also at regular intervals thereafter.

After a few days in the hospital, we took Mom to my sister's home. Mom had her own room in my sister's house. My sisters and I planned a schedule so one of us would be with Mom always. I watched my mother on Mondays, Tuesdays, Wednesdays, and Fridays from 6 am to 5 pm. My sister Janet watched her on the other three days and in the evenings. At the time, little to nothing did I know about opioids, benzodiazepines, cancer, medicine, medical practice, or how Mom was being treated.

Once home, my mother was under the care of the Hospice doctor. The Hospice doctor had not seen my mother. I am not certain what drugs my mother was on in the hospital. Whatever drugs she was on should have been stopped when she went home.

The Hospice nurse came by the house. The nurse told us to give Mom the white pill, Lorazepam, one or two, every four hours, or more often if needed. The nurse told us to give Mom the pink pill, Oxycodone, one or two, every six hours, or more frequently as needed. Oxycodone is an opioid. Opioids do not treat the cause of your pain. Opioids work by blocking receptors in your brain so you do not feel pain.

My mother was not in pain while sitting down. She was only in pain when she stood on her left leg, caused by the tumor in her left hip. Otherwise she was not suffering. Next to my mom's bed was a portable toilet. Mom needed to get from the bed to the toilet. Mom also needed to get into a wheelchair for us to take her for a walk, bring her into the dining area to join in for meals, or into the family room to have some company to watch TV. However, most of the time Mom was in bed.

Mom did not need Oxycodone to sit or lay in bed. She was not in pain then. She could get to the toilet and into the wheelchair, with some pain, without Oxycodone. Mom would have been much better off not taking Oxycodone. At the least, Mom could have taken a tiny dose of Oxycodone on occasion.

She should not have been on a six hour dosing regimen. My mother should have been on a holistic treatment plan for pain management.

Oxycodone and Lorazepam are controlled substances. The nurse cannot prescribe these drugs. Only a doctor can prescribe these drugs. The Hospice doctor prescribed these drugs without seeing my mother. In addition to this being malpractice, and possibly a felony, this is a lack of respect for the patient as an individual.

Issues With Hospice

1. Giving my mother Oxycodone.

2. Irresponsibly prescribing drugs.

3. Prescribing medication without seeing the patient.

4. Not having holistic treatment for pain management.

5. Not having respect for the patient as an individual.

Chapter 8 Radiation Therapy

> When I first moved here and did not know anyone, your mother befriended me. She made me feel welcome.

> ~ Al Lewen

On Thursday, a couple of days after my mother came home from the hospital, we took her to the radiation oncologist to prepare her for radiation therapy. The office was magnificent with an expansive atrium, overly wide hallways, beautiful artwork, and decorations. At the first appointment, the radiation therapist showed us a film of what was going to happen. After the film, she answered questions.

We were in a large room with a long table on which the patient lies. Large, sophisticated space age machines hung over the table. We left Mom with the technician. With the assistance of the machines, the technician marked my mother's body for the radiation therapy that was to take place starting Monday. You leave the marks on your body for the duration of the therapy to properly align the machines. When Mom came out of the technician's office, she was a mess. She was stressed out, did not want to have the radiation therapy, and wanted to go home. We asked her what happened to frighten her but could not get an answer. To me, the people in the radiation oncologist's office were God's healing angels. The machines were a miracle of science. My mother saw a torture chamber.

The consequences of not having the radiation therapy would be disastrous. Cancer loves bones. The tumors would grow fast. The pain would increase. The tumor in her hip would keep her bedridden, a disaster by itself, causing physical and emotional suffering, depression, brittle bones, bed sores, and on and on. The tumor in her back could collapse her spine causing paralysis. She had to have the radiation therapy unless the oncologist's pill Tarceva® worked a miracle, which sometimes happens.

The radiation oncologist came to talk with us. The radiation oncologist said some people get relief quickly, but you should not expect to see results until the end of the second week or later. Eventually, we got Mom to agree to go to ten radiation treatments over the next two weeks.

We took Mom for treatment on Monday, Tuesday and Wednesday. On Thursday, she refused to go. She only went to three of her scheduled ten radiation treatments. By the way, the radiation oncologist's office billed Medicare $21,000 for those four visits. The radiation therapy did not hurt. All my mother had to do was let us drive her to the office and lie on a table for twenty minutes. There were other folks, some older than her, cheerfully coming and going by themselves. One older guy remarked, "Here I am, in and out for my daily dose."

Why was my mother so irrational? At that point, Mom was on three mind altering drugs Escitalopram, Oxycodone, and Lorazepam. She was also taking a number of other medications. Probably the medications were making her crazy.

Back home, I figured Mom would quickly get bored sitting in bed all day. Once she saw she was not dying immediately, I thought she would be forced to accept she was living with cancer. I assumed she would be willing to then see her friends, which would encourage her. She would want to get out of the room and start doing things. This would lead her to take the necessary steps of seeing the oncologist and radiation oncologist.

Thursday was my day off from watching my mother. I watched her during the day on Friday. We had a fight, because I was mad she refused to go back to the radiation oncologist. I did not see her on Saturday and Sunday. On Monday, I realized my mother was never going to get bored sitting in bed. She was never going to want to see her friends. She was never going to accept her situation. My mother was already gone in la la land. She was lying in bed getting high off Oxycodone and Lorazepam, which she later admitted. Only 17 days after her diagnosis, she was a drug addict. Hospice had already effectively killed her.

On Tuesday, in going from the bed to the toilet, I saw my mother put her full weight on her left leg. This was at the end of her Oxycodone cycle, so the Oxycodone was not masking pain. This was the first time she put weight on that leg since going into the hospital. I thought the radiation must have helped.

On Friday, I went into my mother's room to find my mother had gotten a change of clothes. I asked her how she got the clothes. She said she did not know. To get the clothes, she had to have walked a few steps across the room, bent down to open the dresser draws, taken the clothes, closed the drawers, and walked back to her bed. That would have put pressure on her hip and been impossible before. After only three radiation treatments, the pain in her hip was gone.

My mother was cured. If not cured, at least you could say cancer was no longer bothering her. Had my mother not been on drugs, I believe she would have resumed her life then. Only three weeks earlier, my mother was living her life. She was going to lunch with her friends. She was doing things. She could have been doing those things again, even better, because her hip pain was relieved.

Granted, she had been depressed. However, now she knew what the problem was. The tumors were shrunk. She was not in pain. Perhaps she would have accepted her diagnosis and made up her mind to live with her situation. Given something positive to do by adopting a nutritious, anti-cancer diet, and with becoming active and seeing her friends, maybe she would have some hope and feel better about her situation. This pro-active, holistic approach had to be better than what Hospice did. At that point, my mother had won the battle with cancer, for the moment, but Hospice had made her a drug addict.

Issues With Hospice

1. Overmedicating my mother.

2. Turning my mother into a drug addict.

3. Depriving my mother of a chance to face her situation.

4. Depriving my mother of living her life after successful radiation therapy.

Part II Winning the First Battle for My Mother's Life

מוֹדֶה אֲנִי לְפָנֶיךָ מֶלֶךְ חַי וְקַיָּם שֶׁהֶחֱזַרְתָּ בִּי נִשְׁמָתִי בְּחֶמְלָה
רַבָּה אֱמוּ תֶן :

I give thanks to You, King living and enduring, Who mercifully restored my soul unto me, great is Your faithfulness.

~ Modeh Ani, I Give Thanks to You, Jewish blessing upon awakening

Chapter 9 Drug Addiction

וַיְהִי אַחַר הַדְּבָרִים הָאֵלֶּה וְהָאֱלֹהִים נִסָּה אֶת אַבְרָהָם וַיֹּאמֶר אֵלָיו אַבְרָהָם

וַיֹּאמֶר הִנֵּנִי .

And it came to pass after these things that God tested Abraham, and said to him: "Abraham";

And he answered: "Here I am."

~ Genesis 22:1

Everyone that gets a diagnosis of cancer is devastated. They are scared, depressed and feel hopeless. When something terrible happens to you, you go through a process like in grieving. After a while, you have to accept what happened. You have to find a way to live your life. You cannot go to your doctor to get drugs to get you high so you do not have to deal with your situation. Your doctor will not give you drugs for that. Unless you have Hospice treating you. In that case, Hospice will overmedicate you until you lose your mind. Then, you never have to deal with your situation. That is what Hospice did to my mother. Hospice irresponsibly, and illegally, prescribed drugs regardless of consequences.

To recap, the first week, Mom went to the hospital, got her diagnosis, and went home to my sister's house. The second week she had three radiation treatments. By the end of the third week, though the radiation treatment worked, my mother was lying in bed in a stupor.

People get cancer and go on living their life. The cancer, or possibly the treatment, may eventually kill them, but people do not usually drop dead from cancer immediately after their diagnosis. A friend of mine, who is a home care nurse and treats cancer patients, told me her mother had the same diagnosis as Mom. Her mother was told she had weeks to live. She was older than Mom. She did not want aggressive treatment either. She lived for four years and died of something else. That woman lived in Puerto Rico, where they have more healthcare options. She had both an oncologist and a naturopath treating her.

My mother was a fighter. She took care of herself. She was busy from early morning until she pooped out in the evening. She walked a couple miles every morning. She worked in the yard. She went up and down the steps in the house. She went out every day to meet with friends. When she was not running around doing something, she knitted and read. Mom was a practical person. She was the opposite of a procrastinator. She did not let things go. She kept the house immaculate. If something needed doing, she anguished over the thing until the thing got done. Try lying in bed when you are not tired. I did. I was ready to go out of my mind after ten minutes. Knowing my mother, I believe she would have gotten out of bed as soon as she could if she were not on the drugs. As I mentioned earlier, she did get out of bed as soon as I got her off the opioids.

Imagine going into an opium den and finding your mother strung out on a couch. That was what watching my mother was like only those people in the opium den go home after they binge. My mother was home. She was strung out all day long, day after day. I went nuts. I was complaining to everyone, Hospice, family members, and friends. People were saying I was having trouble accepting my mother was dying. They were telling me to go along.

Drugging the patient is the easiest thing to do. People want to believe the easiest thing to do is the right thing to do. My mother could not advocate for herself. She had no one to look out for her, but me. I thought about how Mom acted when one of us were in need. Mom would not succumb to what was going on. If she knew something was wrong, Mom became a terror. One time after the Hospice workers saw my mom, I showed them a picture of my mother when she was in her forties. She looked great. I told them, "She is not a zombie. She is a person, just like you. That is not her in there. She has feelings. She is sociable. You are drugging her into a stupor."

Hospice blamed my mother's mental state on the cancer, saying the cancer may have spread to her brain. They told me I needed to let go. The Hospice people said Mom had weeks to live. They said the cancer had spread throughout her body. They took out Mom's medical chart. They said she had lesions in her organs. They were wrong. There were calcifications, not tumors. Outside her lungs, Mom only had the tumors in her hip and back. Even with this corrected information, Hospice did not change their practices. Incompetence and assuredness often go together. People who are good at what they do, question what they do.

The Hospice nurse came once or twice each week. The nurse said my mother's lungs were clear. She was breathing fine. Her heart was strong. Her vital signs were good. Still Hospice insisted that Mom was on her death bed. My mother was actually kind of healthy. Except she was addicted to Oxycodone and Lorazepam, and of course had lung cancer.

Like many drugs, you develop a tolerance to Oxycodone. You need higher doses of the drug to get the same effect. You quickly develop an addiction to Oxycodone. Oxycodone is a short acting opioid. Oxycodone does not stay in your body long, which is good. The problem is you start to suffer withdrawal symptoms after six hours. Lorazepam has similar issues.

The Hospice people were cavalierly telling us to dispense these drugs. They said to us, "If you need to sleep at night, give her a couple more before you go to bed." Hospice was telling us to drug my mother so we could sleep? I could not believe what I was hearing. Since when do you treat the patient based on the needs of the caretaker? That is medical malpractice. In Fritz Leiber's "My Lady of Darkness", one of the characters tells a tale of a night nurse that worked on a ward for the mentally ill. The nurse was notorious for overmedicating the patients, so she would not have to deal with them. One morning, when the day shift arrived, they found the nurse gone and all the patients dead. That is when I started staying overnight. I did not want my mother overmedicated in the evening. In addition to watching my mom four days a week, from that point on, I watched her every night.

Drug addiction is terrible. My mother had gone through her whole life without being dependent on drugs. At the end of her life, in a matter of a week or so, Hospice addicted my mother, not to one, but to two terrifying drugs. Think about that for yourself. You go through your life a normal, healthy person. You get an awful diagnosis of cancer. Hospice comes in promising to keep you comfortable. The next thing you know, you are a dope addict, like a heroin junkie. With Hospice though, there is no limit to the drugs you get.

For my mother, life became about when she was going to get her pills. She was like Frodo with the Ring of Fire, always seeing the "great pink ball", as she called the Oxycodone pill, in the sky between her eyes. For her, her life had one purpose, to get her next fix. I got a lot of work done during this time. Most of the time, my mother laid in bed semi-conscious. She hardly bothered me. As my mother became more tolerant, she asked for the drugs more frequently. I refused to give her the drugs more frequently than every six hours.

She was not in pain from the cancer, but the drugs were losing their effectiveness in getting her high. She was suffering from drug side effects that caused her pain. She was also suffering withdrawal symptoms at the end of each drug cycle. She started pestering us for drugs hours early. On the table in front of her, I put a little clock, and a paper sign with the time when she was going to get the drugs next. Still, every few minutes she would say, "It is time for my pills now."

By this point, she barely knew who she was. She would call my sister "our friend", because she could not remember Janet's name. She could no longer tell time. She would ask for the drugs literally, every 45 seconds. She would keep that up for three hours, non-stop. I could no longer work. She would try every tactic to get the drugs. She would reason, irrationally of course, accuse, blame, curse, plead, and say anything to get the drugs earlier than scheduled.

I had a girlfriend that called me a bulldog. My girlfriend had said if something was bothering me, I would not let the issue drop. I told Hospice my mother was no longer in pain. She was addicted to the drugs. All her suffering was being caused by her treatment, not the cancer.

When I worked for IBM, I worked on a helpdesk. People called in with their problems. I saw that their problems were solved. I closed over 20,000 problems. When someone reported a problem, we did not consider the problem solved until the customer was satisfied. We have all had bad experiences calling a helpdesk to report a problem. I think helpdesks have gotten a lot better. However, in earlier days, I often felt that the helpdesk treated me as the problem, not what I was reporting. The problem to them was that I was reporting a problem. The sooner the person on the helpdesk got rid of me, the sooner their problem went away.

Hospice behaved in a similar way to those helpdesks. The problem to Hospice was not my mother's drug addiction. The problem was me objecting to what was happening.

Issues With Hospice

1. Not acknowledging their incompetence in misreading my mother's medical reports.

2. Their assuredness in pronouncing how long my mother had to live.

3. Treating patients for the convenience of the caretakers.

4. Going about business as usual, ignoring my mother's drug addiction when I raised the issue.

5. Stealing my mother's mind.

6. Depriving us of a chance to save my mother.

Chapter 10 The Hospice Staff

וְכִתְכֹעַ שׁוֹ ר תִּשְׁמָעוּ

When the shofar sounds, listen!

~ Isaiah 18:3

The Hospice staff that came by the house consisted of a nurse who provided medical care, such as giving medications, listening to the lungs, taking blood pressure and treating sores. Most of the time we had the same nurse. There were healthcare workers that bathed Mom, changed the bed sheets and changed Mom's clothes. A social worker came by, maybe once a month. All of them sometimes brought someone with them that was in training. They were all pleasant, caring people. We liked them all.

They have an emotionally demanding job. They treat people who are dying. They have to see people who are in distress. They have to see families in distress. The end result is death. Thankfully they are willing to do this job. For the months that we were taking care of Mom, I appreciated their caring efforts. They tried to be sensitive to Mom and us. They treated Mom like a dear friend.

My complaints about Hospice are not directed at these folks individually. The healthcare workers played no part in my issues. The nurses and social workers were nice people who believed in what they were doing. Some had lost family members recently, having gone through the experience we were going through. Some started working for Hospice because they had lost a family member previously and they felt Hospice had helped them.

59

Responsibility for my Mom's healthcare fiasco lies with the Hospice doctor and the Hospice system. While I do not blame the nurses and social workers, they were blind to my mother's situation. They were the ones in the room seeing my mother. They were the ones I was ranting and raving to. They were not only blind, they were deaf in the face of my constant criticism. They were the ones who could have made a difference. Yet they insisted they were right without listening to my alarms.

While my mother was sick, there was a 16 year old boy Robert Dentmond that was killed by our local police. The boy had called 911 saying he was going to kill himself. You can listen to his 911 call on YouTube. He sounds like a distraught, polite teenager, saying numerous, "Yes Ma'ams" to the woman taking the call.

Several patrol units confronted the boy. The boy was holding a toy gun that was a replica of an AR-15. On the 911 call the boy said the gun was an M16. The police told the boy to put the gun down, which he did, but then he picked the gun back up. According to the police report, the boy started walking towards the apartment buildings. The police told the boy to put the gun down again or they "would be forced to fire if he continued towards the occupied building while armed." "As a result of Mr. Dentmond's refusal to comply with the directions of Deputies and Officers, lethal force was utilized to stop the threat Mr. Dentmond posed to residents of the complex."

The police report is misleading. Robert Dentmond posed no threat. A correct report would say "lethal force was utilized to stop the threat police mistakenly believed Mr. Dentmond posed to residents". The Sheriff Sadie Darnell said the officers did nothing wrong. The police refuse to take responsibility for their error even when they know the facts.

I was teaching dancing in Hawthorne. I used to drive through a poor neighborhood to get there. One time, the area was cordoned off. There must have been two hundred police officers there. They had two armored vehicles. There was a helicopter overhead. I asked someone what was going on. The police were going into a house to get one guy. The police know who the bad guys are.

This boy Robert Dentmond had no history of violence. The boy had not threatened anyone but himself. The boy had not fired on the police. The boy had not fired the gun. The police could see they were dealing with a teenager. The police knew they were dealing with a boy who had called to say he was going to kill himself not others. I imagine the police could see they were dealing with someone who had no idea how to use a gun. The police could see that the boy did not even know what kind of gun he had. Yet the police did not investigate whether the gun was real, or where this 16 year old might have gotten an AR-15, or if the gun was even loaded.

Why did the police use lethal force? Even if the boy had a real gun, why shoot to kill? There are weapons the police could use to disable the boy, such as a dog. The grand jury report said that the police were too far away to use the dog because the boy could have fired on the dog. Yet that would have told the police whether the gun was real, loaded, and the boy willing and able to shoot. Perhaps a sniper could have shot the gun instead of the boy. What was the hurry to kill the boy?

I have a friend who says, blame the people who trained the officers. Yes, the trainers should be blamed. The Sheriff should be blamed. The system should be blamed. They are all at fault. However, the trainers and the Sheriff were not at the apartment complex that day, the officers were. A police officer, like you and I, is a person. In the end, that person had to take aim at a teenager and pull the trigger. We all know from Nuremberg, you cannot use the defense that you were following orders. You cannot use the defense you were doing what you were trained to do. Your training cannot cover every conceivable circumstance. To me, this is a question of how we value life. If that was your own child, would you shoot him? If not, then do not shoot someone else's child.

Like the Hospice workers that were seeing my mother, these are bad mistakes, mistakes that cause suffering, mistakes that take lives away from people, mistakes you should not, and cannot make. People need to do better. When someone calls 911 and says they are going to shoot themselves, pay attention and help them. Do not murder them. When someone tells you, you are murdering their mother by overdosing her on drugs, pay attention. Stop.

The social worker came to see us. She brought another woman with her who was in training. When one of the Hospice people came to see my mother, whether the nurse or social worker or anyone else that wanted to talk with Mom, I left the room so they could speak freely without my influencing the interaction. Maybe my mother wanted to complain about me. After the social worker spoke with Mom. They asked me how I was doing.

I told them how upset I was. I ranted about how Hospice was drugging my mother into a stupor and all the other things you have read about here. The social worker disagreed with me. She should have listened to what I was telling her. She should have reformed her opinion. Instead, she tried to reform mine.

After the social workers left, Mom said, "The ghouls have come and gone." Mom was still making jokes.

My mother was a charming person. I was always eager for people to meet my parents because they both were so sociable. I could leave anyone alone with either of my parents. My parents would keep them engaged until I got back. No matter how much my mother was suffering, when someone from Hospice came, Mom rose to the occasion. When the doorbell rang, Mom could have been in anguish. Two seconds later, when the Hospice person walked into the room, Mom would sit up, smile, and say, "Nice to see you." When they would ask how she was doing, even though she was complaining moments before, Mom would say to the Hospice person, "I am fine." Mom always wanted to make the people she interacted with feel good.

A couple of Hospice people visited with Mom. After talking with my mother, they said to me that my mother "had made her peace and was ready to die."

I was upset. I told them, "That was completely wrong. She has not made her peace with dying. She is depressed. She is scared. She feels hopeless. She does not want to die. She does not want to deal with her situation. What she wants is not to have cancer. That is very different from making your peace with dying."

They insisted I was wrong.

I said, "She is sitting right there. Ask her."

They asked her.

My mother said, "He is not wrong."

That should have woken up Hospice to an opposite course of action. That should have told Hospice that they have a patient who should not be under their care. My mother needed to have her emotional needs treated, possibly through professional care, possibly through a support group. She was not ready to die. None of that mattered to Hospice. Hospice had an agenda to move, by which I mean kill, my mother through the system as quickly as possible, regardless of what the actual situation was in front of them.

Issues With Hospice

1. Not listening to the patient.

2. Their determination in sticking to their agenda.

Chapter 11 Family and Friends

בָּרוּךְ אַתָּה ו׳ אֱלֹהֵינוּ וֵאלֹהֵי אֲבוֹתֵינוּ ... גּוֹמֵל חֲסָדִים טוֹבִים

Blessed are You Hashem our God and God of our fathers, ... Who bestows loving kindness

~ Amidah, Jewish service central prayer

My mother said she did not want to see any visitors or talk to anyone on the phone. My sister commented that our neighbor Magaret Thaler did the same thing when she was diagnosed with lung cancer. Janet said Margaret was always so put together, she probably did not want people to see her ill. I suspect Margaret was overmedicated too.

Relatives came to visit Mom anyway. My mother's brother Saul had three children Michael, Lynne and Jay. They are the same ages as my sisters and me. Right after my mother got diagnosed, my sister was supposed to meet Michael and Lynne in Fort Myers for vacation. Instead, Michael and Lynne drove up to see us. My sister did not want to tell my mother ahead of time for fear my mother would get too stressed, but I thought I knew Mom better. I told Mom they were coming. She was fine. My mother was their only aunt. They cried when they saw her.

Most of the relatives my parents' age were either no longer living or too old to travel. My Dad's youngest cousins Bill and Leah flew in from Washington, DC. Mom and Leah got on so well, people would think my mother and Leah were related, but Bill was my Dad's blood relative. The women were in-laws. Bill and Leah visited with Mom for a while. Mom summoned her strength as best she could to participate. The visit was good for all of us, but Mom was not herself, not because of the cancer. Mom was on too many drugs to do much more than smile and nod. The drugs made Mom so uncomfortable in so many ways, she could not sustain the effort for long.

My dad's brother, my Uncle Jerry and Aunt Diane and their children, my cousins Michael, Leah and Mandy, and their families drove over from Jacksonville for the day. Michael and Leah had flown in from New York. The visit was good for us. By then, my mother was so gone on drugs, she could only take a visit for a few minutes before losing concentration. Michael and Lynne came back with their families. The same situation played out. Mom was so drugged, she could barely interact with anyone.

Mom's friends called Janet and I regularly. Talking to people of my mother's generation was markedly different, more satisfying and more comforting, than talking to people of my generation. With age comes wisdom. Our society should value that wisdom more. You feel alone when tragedy arrives. The more people you talk with, the more you see how everyone has some story of grief.

Amy, a friend in my dance classes, has a story suitable for a novel. She was abandoned by her mother as a child. Her father moved them in with his parents. Her father passed away when she was eight. Her grandmother got sick. Her grandfather and she took care of her grandmother until her grandmother passed away. As a teenager, her grandfather started doing poorly. Social services tried to take her away, but her grandfather kept them together. At 16 her grandfather passed away. She was put in foster care. At 17 she moved out on her own. Today she is as sweet a person as you would want to know.

Amy used to work for Hospice. She was one of the first people I found that expressed the same things I did. She quit Hospice because of the same abuses I am describing here. The more people you talk to, the more you find stories similar to your own.

My parents moved our family to Gainesville in 1971. The synagogue, Congregation B'nai Israel, was in an old church that backed up to our neighborhood. My parents joined the synagogue and were active members since. Last year my mother paid $600 for our dues. Throughout the year, for each request, she made a donation, on relatives' yahrzeits (anniversary of death), honoring the rabbi, honoring a member, a fundraiser, the sisterhood, someone passing away and so on. She gave another $2,000 in donations.

Soon after we moved to Gainesville, the synagogue moved to a new location, one mile to the west. My parents were on the building committee. Phil Emmer, a member and local real estate developer, with great foresight, provided a fantastic five acre piece of property in the best location. We could never have gotten such a great spot at that late date. In my high school there were two Jewish girls, my sister and Phil's daughter Jodi, a good friend of my sister's. Sadly Jodi passed away young.

Synagogue members and other friends could not have been more supportive of us. They asked after our welfare, listened kindly and gave us needed hugs. They sent cards, flowers and gifts throughout my mother's illness. We read all the letters to my mother. We replied to none of them.

My parents were not religious, but I am. They went to synagogue occasionally. I attend every week. At services, during the Torah reading, that is the Five Books of Moses, we do a prayer for healing called the Mi Shebeirach, which means "May the One Who blessed". Before the blessing, in turn, you say out loud the name of the person in need of healing. You say the name in Hebrew if you can, but as child of their mother instead of the usual father. My mother's name is "Edis bat Ida", which is Yiddish not Hebrew. I did the same for my dad. His name was "Schmiel Mendel ben Berta", which is also Yiddish. Neither one had a Hebrew name. Debbie Friedman wrote a beautiful, powerful, moving song "Mi Shebeirach", that many synagogues, ours included, sing during this portion of the service. You can look this song up. This would be worth your time.

Issues With Hospice

1. Depriving my mother's friends of seeing my mother.

2. Depriving us, her family, of spending meaningful time with her.

3. Depriving my mother of spending meaningful time with family and friends.

Chapter 12 Keep Comfortable

הַשְׁכִּיבֵנ וּ ' אֱלֹהֵינוּ לְשָׁלוֹנ , וְהַעֲמִידֵנוּ מַלְכֵּנוּ לְחַיִּינ .

Lay us down to sleep, Hashem our God in peace, and raise us up, our King, to life.

~ Hashkeveinu, Jewish Prayer

Opioids have bad side effects. You have opioid receptors throughout your body. Opioids negatively affect other organs besides your brain. Opioids cause constipation. They put your bowels to sleep. Your bowels stop working. Food stops moving through them.

My Mom had cancer, but cancer was not causing her suffering. As noted earlier, Mom did not need to be on Oxycodone or Lorazepam. Her hip was no longer hurting her, yet she was lying in bed in a drugged stupor for two months. All her suffering was caused by her medical treatment from Hospice. I kept careful track of everything that my mother complained of. I questioned her in depth about what hurt, where, how much, and how often. I tried to identify each pain and their cause so we would know how to treat them. Mom was suffering from four pains.

The first was from constipation and all the associated discomfort. My mother stopped being able to move her bowels because of the Oxycodone. She was suffering terrible pain in her bowels. My sister dis-impacted my mother by hand. That means pulling out the poop with your fingers. My sister the doctor said to me, "At work we say, monkey see, monkey do, monkey teach. Next time it is your turn."

We had to give my mother enemas. This was awful for her, because she could not sit on the toilet for long. She had to lay on her side waiting for the enema to work, which they failed to do as often as they were successful. Mom dreaded all of this. She was so out of her mind, she insisted that one of us go to the bathroom for her. She thought that if we went, she would not have to. She would say to my brother-in-law Steve, "Will you go upstairs for me." There were no stairs. She was asking him to go to the bathroom so she would get relief from the constipation. The constipation was constant for two months. My mother suffered from constipation pain the whole time. Starting with the third week, for the next five weeks, Hospice was literally giving my mother Oxycodone to treat the pain Mom had from the constipation that the Oxycodone was causing.

The second pain was the withdrawal symptoms that she suffered at the end of her cycles for Oxycodone and Lorazepam, As she neared the end of the cycle for each drug, she got fidgety. The discomfort was different for each. She had various types of anguish from sweats, to pain all over, anxiety, paranoia and more. At the end of her Lorazepam cycle, she would say, "Do not leave me." When we assured her, she would say, "You swear you will not leave me?" She would ask us to get into bed with her. The bed was the size of a twin bed, with rails.

The third pain my mother had was nausea from all the drugs she was taking. For the nausea, Hospice had her on yet another drug Ondansetron, brand name Zofran. Note that these were not all the drugs she was on. There were drugs for acid reflux Omeprazole, brand name Prilosec, which she did not need when she was eating the diet I had her on. There were also a couple of different pills for constipation, which did not work.

The fourth pain my mother had was from a bed sore, a small hole on her coccyx. This was caused by her being bedridden by the drugs. The bed sore hurt her a lot. This was a scary development, because bed sores can quickly get worse and are hard to heal. People die from bed sores. Hospice gave us good instructions to treat the bed sore. Mom was still getting in and out of bed to use the toilet so she was moving around which is crucial to treating the sore. We put cream on the sore. Fortunately, the sore healed over.

On top of the various pains, she was a drug addict for two drugs. She had a constant craving to get high. Opioids cause you to lose your appetite. Cancer causes you to lose your appetite too. You see pictures of heroin addicts who are emaciated so you know that opioids do not need help from cancer to stop you from eating. My mother was not eating much and not exercising at all. Lying in bed and not eating for two months ruins your body. She lost all her muscle. Lying in bed your bones can become brittle and break from simply rolling over. As far as we know, she did not break any bones.

Two months into my mother's illness Mom had suffered every day, not from the cancer but from her treatment. If my mother did not have me advocating for her and had I not written this book, nobody would have known. Hospice would have said they kept my mother as comfortable as possible. Everyone would have blamed, they did blame, the cancer for Mom's suffering.

Issues With Hospice

1. Shutting down my mother's digestive system.

2. Keeping my mother bedridden.

3. Causing my mother to lose all her muscle.

4. Causing my mother unnecessary pain.

Chapter 13 Good News

הָפַכְתָּ מִסְפְּדִי לְמָחוֹל לִי פִּתַּחְתָּ שַׂקִּי וַתְּאַזְּרֵנִי שִׂמְחָה :

You have turned my mourning into dancing;

You have loosened my sackcloth and girded me with joy;

~ David, Psalm 30

My youngest sister Randi came back into town to give Janet and I a break from watching Mom. Randi did not have the experience the other two of us had in forestalling Mom's request for drugs. By the time Randi went home, after a week, my mother was asking for the drugs every two hours.

The next day I refused to give my mother the drugs as frequently as she wanted. I left the room for a little while. When I came back, my mother had walked across the room, gotten the Oxycodone and Lorazepam out of their child proof bottles, taken the pills, and gotten back in bed. Mom had not walked since the time she got her clothes on her own a few weeks earlier. She never could open child proof bottles. Shows you what motivation can do.

We moved the drugs out of Mom's room. Janet woke up to Mom's addiction and started cooperating in reducing Mom's dose. I finally had some help in getting my mother straightened out. We started weaning my mother off the Oxycodone. We started lengthening the time between doses to get her up to six hours again. Janet would give my mother a placebo which would often placate Mom. See, there are other ways to treat pain. Instead of giving my mother Oxycodone and Lorazepam at the same time, we split them up, each one every three hours in the hope that would stall her. We were still giving her Escitalopram.

My poor mother was suffering terribly from these drugs. Imagine having multiple drug addictions and not have your cravings satisfied. You might think not giving her the drugs as frequently as she wanted was cruel, but you could not give her drugs as often as she wanted, because she had developed a tolerance and wanted the drugs more and more frequently. This is what had happened with Randi. We had seen the result of that experiment.

Mom was out of her mind. She pitifully would ask, "Will pressing the button help me?" My brother-in-law had given her a doorbell she could ring to call for us. She would ring the doorbell to ask for her drugs. She had associated the feeling of getting high with ringing the doorbell. Sometimes Mom would ask, "Will drinking water from the red cup help me?" She also associated the feeling the drugs gave her with the red cup because that is what she drank water out of to wash down the pills.

The drugs caused a host of tortures. We could not tell what drug was doing what to her. We stopped giving her the Escitalopram. We have no idea what good or bad the Escitalopram ever did.

Sunday night through Thursday morning, I was now watching my mother the entire time for all but a few hours in the evening. I stopped giving her the Oxycodone altogether. That night and the next, she had withdrawal symptoms and vomited both nights. The day after she seemed fine. She did not remember what happened to her. That day, Janet said she talked to the pharmacist at her work, who said we should take Mom down to two Oxycodone a day this week, one a day the next week, and then stop. I was happy for the support, though I commented again on how people were treating Mom without seeing her. I told Janet that I thought Mom had suffered the worst of her withdrawal symptoms the night before and she did not need Oxycodone any more. Janet did not give my mother any more Oxycodone.

The day after that my mother woke up, got up, started eating, started pooping, and started walking. When Hospice came by they could not believe what they were seeing. The Hospice healthcare worker exclaimed, "She is walking!"

Had I went along with Hospice's protocol, I believe my mother would have been dead within the first few weeks under Hospice's care. Two months after her diagnosis, my mother was almost a person again. She was talking. We were doing some things with her like reading to her. I took her outside in the wheelchair. I started getting Mom to exercise in bed. I started getting her to use the walker. One time while I was tucking her in, Mom said to me in a childlike voice, "You would make a good daddy."

Mom was still on Lorazepam. Mom was not herself in terms of her mental faculties. Her personality had somewhat returned. She was her cheerful self when not suffering from Lorazepam side effects. She did not seem depressed anymore. She seemed to have accepted her situation. I encouraged some friends of hers to call. She spoke to them for the first time. Diane Heaney, my mother's good friend of 40 years, came by for a visit. This was the one time Mom saw any of her friends.

Mom stopped using the buzzer to call us. Instead she yelled for us when she wanted something. She started getting up out of bed on her own. She would get on and off the portable toilet by herself when no one was in the room. She walked across the room to get her clothes. A few times she walked out of her room into the hallway looking for one of us. A couple of times she fell. She yelled for help. I was sleeping in the room next door. One time my nephew Josh heard her and

Josh woke me up. One time I heard her. Both times I found her on the floor. She did have a bruise on the right side of her face. Otherwise she seemed alright.

Mom was showing good signs. When you are caring for someone, even when caring for yourself, if you are doing more things than you were before, you are getting better. After two months, Mom had turned around. Mom was doing more. I had hopes. I wrote an email titled "Good News" to family members who had come to visit Mom when she was a zombie. I told them for the moment, Mom was doing better. Whatever the future might bring, we had a good week.

Part III Losing the War With Doctor Death

A person's system of elimination is essential to his well-being.

~ Rabbi Schneur Zalman of Liadi, Alter Rebbe's Shulcan Aruch

Chapter 14 Nutrition

פּוֹתֵחַ אֶת יָדֶךָ וּמַשְׂבִּיעַ לְכָל חַי רָצוֹן :

You open Your hand, and satisfy the wants of all living.

~ Jewish prayer

When Mom was in the hospital, I went into Mom's room to find her eating dinner. The hospital had brought her beef stroganoff which is beef with noodles, and a dessert of ice cream. Mom was not eating much, but I was distressed about the food she was eating. Mom had been diagnosed with cancer. I expected her to be on the most nutritious, anti-cancer diet. Here she was served three foods that cause inflammation, suppress the immune system, and fuel cancer. No doubt Mom selected that dinner from a menu, but I was put off by the lack of attention to nutrition by the medical staff. Mom was in the cancer ward. On the wall by the nurses station was a poster of what to eat for someone that had cancer which was not those foods. You hear of people who get cancer, and I have known some, who put themselves on the healthiest regime they can with the most nutritious diet. You hear them say, "I feel better now than I have in my whole life. The only problem is I have cancer." I expected the same for my mother.

I am not a professional researcher, nor do I treat cancer patients. I do not know for a fact what food causes what effect. I generally do not read the source research. What I do read, and I read a lot, are the people that read the research. The information I find most convincing is that people in non-Westernized societies infrequently die of cancer and heart disease. Westernized societies have more causes of, and less protections against, cancer and heart disease. We do not have a good relationship between our environment, including our food supply, that creates these diseases, and our medical system that treats the diseases. There is a cure for heart disease, eating healthy, or better yet, living healthy. The same cure may be available for cancer. Yet our system makes eating healthy, and living healthy, almost impossible. I stopped at a rest station on the Florida Turnpike. The place was packed. People were eating burgers, fries, pizza, and a few, pesticide-laden salads. There was not one thing to buy that was healthy. I brought my own food, but for a normal person, everything they could purchase to eat promoted cancer or heart disease or both.

How does cancer get you? You are living your life, one cell mutates into cancer and then you are dead? Is that how cancer works? Some people say that everyone may have cancer cells, but your immune system cleans them up. You die from cancer when your immune system cannot remove the cancer cells. Your immune system, and by immune system I mean all your body's defenses, protects you from cancer. The healthier your body, the more protection you have from cancer.

Nutrition is crucial to maintaining your health. Nutrition supports all your body's functions. Good nutrition strengthens your immune system. Good nutrition enhances your mood. You feel better when you eat nutritiously. Your body does not function well with poor nutrition. Poor nutrition weakens your immune system. You feel worse when you do not eat nutritiously.

Good nutrition can fight cancer directly. Many foods inhibit cancer growth. On the other side, many foods promote cancer growth. In simplest terms, natural foods are good. Unnatural foods are bad. Why? Because of millions of years of adaption to the natural environment. There are countless chemical reactions taking place in your body. Sugar is good for you when eaten in a complex of other nutrients like an apple. Your body evolved to eat fruit in all of fruit's biologic complexity. Sugar is not good when extracted from an apple and mixed with water to make apple juice. Your body does not know how to respond to sugar in a form that does not exist in nature.

There is a lot of information online. Search for any food with the word "cancer". You will get numerous articles telling you if that food inhibits or promotes cancer. The articles usually have linked reference studies. There are many foods that have been shown to fight cancer. There are certain foods that cancer loves, in particular, refined carbohydrates, which turn into sugar without the nutritional benefits of whole foods. Tumor growth is fueled by sugar. Other particularly bad foods are non-organic meat, chicken, farm-raised fish, and non-organic dairy, possibly because of the growth hormones, anti-biotics, the bad fat they contain caused by the animals' diets, pesticides, and herbicides, or any number of other factors due to the unnatural conditions in which they are processed.

A lot of the problem is the interaction with your microbiome. Termites cannot digest wood. Microbes in their gut digest the wood for them. Cows cannot digest grass. Microbes digest the grass for the cow. We are the same way. The microbes do more than aid digestion. Researchers have identified hundreds of genes that interact with your microbiome. Again, in simplest terms, bad microbes release compounds that promote cancer growth. Good microbes release compounds that inhibit cancer growth. You want to feed the good microbes and starve the bad microbes. That means eating mostly vegan and avoiding refined carbohydrates and bad fats.

Cancer cells are highly active, more active than most normal cells. Cancer cells are like Audrey II in "Little Shop of Horrors" constantly demanding, "Feed me." The results of my mom lying in bed for two months were mostly bad. The one good thing is that low calorie diets inhibit tumor growth. While Mom was losing her muscles, she may have also been shrinking her tumors.

I have been health conscious since I was a teenager. From the time I was in college, I have been improving my diet. Recently, my doctor was concerned about my blood pressure and wanted to put me on a drug. I told him I would fix my blood pressure with diet and exercise, which I did.

My dad told me, "60 is not like 50. At 50 I felt strong. I could do anything. At 60, I did not feel too good." I was in good shape at 50. Approaching 60, I feel even stronger. I tried to improve my dad's diet. My parents resented my interference. My dad continued to dip his bread in chicken fat. The last few years he was on so much blood pressure medication, he had trouble staying awake during the day. He died at 76. I know now that a vegetarian diet has been proven to reverse clogged arteries. Had the doctors told this to my dad, he may have lived another ten years and felt better for twenty.

Since living with my mother, bit by bit, Mom had been coming around to my diet, which was mostly organic vegan. Mom had a friend that said she was allergic to tomatoes. The friend said that she could not even touch a tomato without breaking out in a rash. I suspected Mom's friend was allergic to the pesticides. I told Mom to give her friend our organic tomatoes. The friend was able to eat our organic tomatoes without a problem. The friend started buying organic tomatoes for herself. Before Mom's diagnosis, Mom was already buying all organic fruits and vegetables, just like me.

For the most part, we had stopped bringing into the house refined carbohydrates like cookies, cakes, ice cream, and bread. I would rather go out for a $5 ice cream cone, than buy two-for-one gallons of ice cream for $4 from the grocery store and bring them home. If you do, you end up eating the ice cream instead of meals. Mom loved meat and sweets. She ate as badly as anyone when she went out with her friends. In the house, she was mostly eating my healthy diet.

I spoke to Hospice about nutrition, but they had no interest. They said what my mother ate does not matter. She only needed calories. They were fine with giving her ice cream or anything else.

In Ft. Lauderdale on an occasion, I was with some people and we saw a mangy raccoon picking through some garbage. The pitiful appearing animal looked malnourished. Another time in Ft. Lauderdale at a city nature preserve on a small island, we saw a group of handsome looking raccoons, large, muscular, with beautiful shiny coats of fur and proud bearings. These raccoons looked well fed. We all know animals are strong and healthy when they are well fed. Animals are weak and raggedy when malnourished. Same for plants. If you want your plants to grow well, give them the right conditions with proper nutrients. Funny how so many of us do not think of people responding in the same way to nutrition.

For the four days of the week that I watched my mother, I fed her most of her meals. Mom often resisted what I gave her, but I gave her the best food. I bought all organic fruits and vegetables. I bought the highest quality supplements. Everything I gave her was reported to reduce inflammation, strengthen the immune system, inhibit cancer growth, shrink tumors and block growth of new blood vessels to the tumors. I made Mom a delicious pureed cauliflower, broccoli, leek soup with turmeric and garlic, five of the top cancer fighting vegetables. All the food I made her was like that, organic, healthy, homemade and delicious, apple-pear sauce, avocado chocolate mousse, granola with fresh fruit. I served her food beautifully garnished on small plates, as taste is influenced by appearance. She liked all of these things. She made them herself at home. Now, she objected to them irrationally. Again, I suspect the drugs.

My mother was like a hostile witness at a trial. She resisted the food and supplements I gave her. When I was not feeding her, she ate the worst foods: non-organic animal products such as meat and dairy; sugar products such as refined carbohydrates, ice cream, cookies and bread; and the worst of both worlds, pizza. These foods are reported to cause inflammation, weaken the immune system, and accelerate cancer growth. My mother needed calories, but giving her a bagel with cream cheese was feeding the tumors, not her. The problem was I had no one on my side. The other caretakers, Hospice included, were nutrition ignorant. Most had not taken a class on nutrition or read the first thing online.

I was on board with my mother declining chemotherapy. Fine, if that was what she wanted. Let us then try an experiment giving her the best nutrition and see how that affected her health. If everything she put in her mouth was reported to kill cancer, I would have liked to have seen how much better she would have done. There are people who have reported successful results fighting cancer with diet.

I would like to address two more points about nutrition, first that people choose to eat the foods that are bad for them. Second that giving them nutritious foods is depriving them of some happiness, because nutritious foods do not taste as good. For the first, in experiments you can find online, a rat will choose cocaine over food and sugar over cocaine. That a person chooses to eat foods that are addictive is not a choice. Across a population there is a gradient of how much bad food people eat. You can say individuals can influence where they fall on that curve, but the curve is determined by the food supply. The food supply in the United States is compromised. With the choices people have, many will eat too much food that is bad for them. For the second, once you detox from the conventional food supply, there is nothing better than fresh fruits and vegetables. Healthy foods taste better and make you feel better.

My mother had reflux for the last decade. When she went to sleep, she propped herself up to avoid the reflux. She was taking Prilosec to control the reflux. She was still taking Prilosec when she had cancer. When I started feeding her, her reflux went away. She did not need Prilosec. I did not give her refined carbohydrates. I did not give her meat either, except occasionally an organic egg and rarely some small pieces of organic, kosher chicken breast. Once she stopped eating sugar, and by sugar I mean refined carbohydrates, her reflux went away. There is support for this outcome online.

She also seemed to do better overall. When she was eating the healthy food I gave her, she had less pain, she was nauseous less, and she did not react as badly at the end of her drug cycles. To me, she clearly felt better when she ate better. The opposite happened as well. Whenever I was not taking care of her, she seemed to have gotten worse. I think she did worse because of the unhealthy food and additional drugs she got from others.

That I felt compelled to include a chapter on nutrition, something that is as basic as the need for clean air and water, is a condemnation of our medical system.

Issues With Hospice

1. Lack of respect for nutrition.

Chapter 15 Lorazepam

בְּיָדוֹ אַפְקִיד רוּחַ .
ו ' לִי וְלֹא אִירָא .

In his hand, I safeguard my spirit.
Hashem is for me and I will not be afraid.

~ Adon Olam, Lord of the Universe, Jewish
liturgical song

Lorazepam

A sedative. Brand name Ativan. Elderly patients are more
likely to have unwanted effects.

Can cause abdominal bleeding, anxiety, confusion,
constipation, depression, disorientation, difficulty
concentrating, hallucinations, impaired judgment, loss of
appetite, lower back or side pain, memory problems,
muscle weakness, nausea, pain all over, paranoia, suicidal
ideation, and withdrawal symptoms.

Use with opioids may result in profound sedation,
respiratory depression, coma, and death.

Once my mother was off Oxycodone, I set about weaning her
off Lorazepam.

In college, I took the hardest undergraduate curriculum of anyone I know. I took the full pre-med curriculum. After my junior year, I had enough credits to graduate with a major in chemistry. I graduated after my senior year with a bachelor's degree in mathematics. I had enough credits for a minor in computer science.

In Chemistry's Quantitative Analysis lab, you measure how much of particular substances are in a solution. Each lab was worth 50 points. You got the full 50 points if you got the correct result. The closer you got, the more points you got. You got a minimum of 5 points for doing the lab even if your result was completely wrong.

In the lab, the first thing you do is wash your beaker. You use a metal tong to place your beaker in the dryer. You then weigh the empty beaker on a scale. You must not touch your beaker, because the weight of the oil from your fingerprint will skew the results. That is how sensitive chemistry is.

You pour the solution in question into your beaker, weighing again, so you know how much solution there is. You then drop another liquid via a pipette, one drop at a time, into the solution. You must count the exact number of drops. At some point, after one particular drop, your solution will change colors, or a substance will precipitate out, or some other effect will happen. You use the number of drops to calculate the result. Just one drop change makes all the difference. That is how sensitive chemistry is.

I got a B in Quantitative Analysis. I got 100s on all the tests. I got 5 points for all the labs. I could do the calculations, but I was useless in the lab. When dropping drops from the pipette into the beaker, you are supposed to count one-by-one, like 1, 2, 3, ..., 151, 152, 153. Instead, I let the pipette run. I would count 20, 40, 60, ... My results were worthless. I had no patience for chemistry's sensitivity.

The medical industry casually dispenses chemicals to people, without seeing them (the Hospice doctor had not seen my mother), without knowing what is going on with the chemistry inside their body, and with far less accuracy than I had in my chemistry labs. If only their results were as useless as mine, but no, their results were horrendous.

Lorazepam is a tranquilizer. My mother should never have been on this drug. There are reports that this drug is not supposed to be given to elderly people. In any case, according to many sources, you should never take this drug for more than two weeks. My mother had been taking this drug every few hours for two months.

Lorazepam is a benzodiazepine. Like opioids, benzodiazepines work by inhibiting the brain's sensors. Benzodiazepines block neurons from giving the brain information about the world. This is supposed to cause the brain to calm down.

Like nearly all drugs, you develop a tolerance. You need more of the drug to get the same effect. Benzodiazepines soon stop working. You then need the drug to keep from going through withdrawal. The withdrawal symptoms for benzodiazepines are bad. The withdrawal symptoms include paranoia, fear, anxiety, sweats, and pain all over. My poor mom suffered from all of them.

Benzodiazepines are harder to get off of than opioids. You cannot suddenly stop taking benzodiazepines like you can with some opioids. With opioids, after the initial withdrawal, you do not suffer more withdrawal symptoms. With benzodiazepines, if you suddenly stop, you continue to suffer withdrawal symptoms which can get worse. You have to slowly reduce the dosage to get off benzodiazepines. Dr. Heather Ashton, who ran a drug recovery clinic in England, developed a method for tapering people off benzodiazepines.

I used the Ashton Method to assist in getting Mom off Lorazepam.

I created a spreadsheet that calculated the amount of Lorazepam in Mom's system based on the half-life of the drug. With the spreadsheet, I could see relatively the high amount of the drug in her system when she got her dose and the low amount at the end of her cycle. In this way, I could wean her off the drug by lengthening the time between dosages. As the time between dosages grew longer, Mom became more coherent. When the dosage intervals exceeded 12 hours, Mom had some moments of lucidity before experiencing withdrawal symptoms. During one of those moments, Mom pitifully said to me, "I do not want all this stuff in my brain." Within an hour of that, she was suffering from withdrawal symptoms. As usual, she started asking for the drug.

After a few weeks, I had gotten her intervals down to the smallest dose once or twice a day. In retrospect, I should have stopped giving her the drug then and there. She would have been drug free for the first time since being diagnosed with cancer. Her head would have cleared. We could have seen what was going on with her. I may have been able to get my mother to fire Hospice. That was not to be. The Hospice doctor intervened. There would be no saving my mother under the Hospice doctor's watch. The Hospice doctor was determined to see my mother dead as soon as possible.

Issues With Hospice

1. Giving my mother Lorazepam.

Chapter 16 Doctor Death

הַרַ ים וְהַמָּ וֶת נָ תִּ י לְפָ יִךְ הַבְּרָ ה וְהַקְּלָ ה
וּבָחַרְתָּ בַּחַ ים

Life and death I have set before you, blessings and curses. Choose life.

~ Deuteronomy 30:19

The Hospice nurse came by. My mother complained of pain. My mother had a pain in her right hip and at times she hurt all over. The nurse blamed cancer. When you have cancer, for every pain you have, you jump to the conclusion that the cancer has spread and is causing you the new pain. Cancer does not work that way. Rogue cancer cells have a difficult time finding a new place in which to settle. Most of the time, conditions are not ideal in most parts of your body for the cancer cells. Your immune system is on patrol and eliminates the cancer cells that are migrating from the source tumor. This makes sense. Tumors shed cells. If cancer could easily metastasize to a new location, once you had one tumor, you would quickly have tumors all over. In most cases, that is not what happens.

The pain in my mother's right hip was probably a bruise from when she fell. This illustrates another problem with using Hospice. With the proper test, you can see if the cancer had spread to another location. Once you are with Hospice, Hospice will not run those tests. They treat your symptoms, without knowing the cause.

Pain all over is a withdrawal symptom of Lorazepam. Mom only had that pain near the end of her Lorazepam cycle.

The nurse wanted to put my mother on Methadone. Janet asked me what I thought of putting my mother on Methadone. I was completely against giving my mother Methadone. My sister was in favor.

Once off the Oxycodone, I had asked my mother about going to see the oncologist. I was not seeing any signs of the cancer having advanced. I wanted to switch Mom from Hospice to the oncologist, who I thought would give better care. The oncologist could run tests. We could find out what was going on with Mom's cancer. We could see if the tumors progressed, stayed the same or had regressed. They could take another biopsy. We could find out what my mother actually had. We could see if she was a candidate for Tarceva®. I wanted to put her on an anti-cancer diet. I thought there was a possibility of her improving. Others have.

Mom continued to refuse to see the oncologist. I was still mad at my mom about that. I said to Janet, "Ask Mom if she wants to go on Methadone. She wants to be her own doctor."

We went in to see Mom. Janet explained what Methadone was. Janet asked Mom if she wanted to be on Methadone. Mom said she did not want to take Methadone. "That drug sounds scary," Mom said. A sentiment you would expect from someone who wants to live, not from someone who has made their peace with dying. The Hospice nurse said they were not ready to prescribe Methadone for my mother anyway.

Randi came back to town to watch Mom. She did not want to be left out. When I watched my mother, she got better. When my sisters watched Mom, she got worse. That is because they gave her more drugs, worse nutrition, and did not holistically treat her. By the end of the week with Randi, Mom was complaining of pain. These were the same pains she had been having, the bruise in her hip and the withdrawal symptoms from the Lorazepam.

The withdrawal symptoms from Lorazepam could get bad. Janet called my mother's reaction "sun-downing" because Janet associated Mom going crazy with evening coming on. Janet's bedtime was 8 pm because she got up early. When Mom was demanding in the evenings, Janet was too tired to deal with Mom. When that happened, Janet would call me to come by early to take care of Mom in the evening.

I could calm Mom down treating her holistically. I would come into Mom's room and find the overhead fan spinning, making noise, creating flickering lights and shadows, and blowing things about. The TV would be on some loud show. The room would be messy. Mom and her bedding would be in disarray. I would turn off the fan, turn off the harsh lights, put on a soft light, shut off the TV, put on meditative music, organize the room, and straighten Mom and her bedding. I would talk to her calmly, telling her everything was going to be alright. I treated her holistically without giving her medication. She relaxed and felt better.

One day when both my sisters were with my mother, my mother complained of pain. Without Oxycodone, my sisters did not know what to do when Mom got stressed out. They had no pill to give Mom, so they called the Hospice doctor. Then they called me and told me the doctor was over. Nothing worse could have happened.

I was in the room with Doctor Death and my mother. The doctor did a cursory examination. She listened to my mother's lung for no more than five seconds. The doctor was talking with my mother asking her if she was in pain. My mother said she was.

I told Doctor Death how I got my mother off Oxycodone. How difficult that was. How much better Mom was doing. I told her how I was weaning Mom off Lorazepam. I told Doctor Death the pain my mother was suffering from was caused by the Lorazepam withdrawal and that pain goes away. I told Doctor Death the cancer was not causing Mom pain. I told her how the radiation therapy worked and Mom could stand on her leg. I told her Mom was not asking for the drugs to relieve pain from the cancer. I told her Mom was asking for the drugs to get high. That giving my mother drugs for her drug addiction was wrong.

Doctor Death was unmoved. After all that we had been through, while sitting there in front of me, after all that I told her, Doctor Death gave my mother an Oxycodone. As my mother drifted off in a stupor, my mother smiled and said, "The golden pill."

I pointed at my mother when Mom said that. I said to Doctor Death, "You see, she wants the drugs to get high, not for pain."

Doctor Death did not care.

My mother got stressed when we argued in front of her. Doctor Death and I left my mother's room. We met with my sisters in the family room to discuss my mother's treatment. Of all the people I met, those most determined to finish what they were doing, those most committed to terminating my mother and ignoring the situation in front of them, the nurse was second, but Doctor Death was far and away first. Like the White Witch from Narnia, the doctor was determined not to let my mother slip through Hospice's grasp and possibly get better. To Doctor Death, my mother must remain on a steady, downward spiral into oblivion. If my mother's body would not cooperate due to my intervention, Doctor Death would take matters into her own hands to force the issue. Doctor Death wanted to put my mother on Methadone.

I objected.

Doctor Death said, "Your mother does not have months to live, she has days to weeks. She will be dead in three weeks."

Had I not been there, I am sure my mother would have been dead in three weeks following Doctor Death's protocol. I asked, "How do you know that? From the examination you just did?"

Doctor Death said, "No, from her report."

I was put off. I asked, "From the report Mom had when she was first in the hospital over two months ago?"

Doctor Death said, "Yes."

I said, "That means you thought she was going to die three weeks after she got out of the hospital and she is still here."

Doctor Death acknowledged that was true. She said, "Your mother has cancer throughout her body."

I said, "No, she does not. Aside from her lungs, she only has a tumor in her left hip and her back. Those have been treated with radiation. Mom responded really well and they are not bothering her." I asked the doctor to look in the report.

Doctor Death reviewed the report. She acknowledged that Mom did not have cancer throughout her body. Outside her lungs, that Mom only had the tumors in her hip and back. Doctor Death did not care. This doctor was not incompetent. This doctor was one smart lady. This was not like the nurse who failed to read the report for herself or understand what she read. This was merciless, brutal arrogance. Any normal person would be horrified making an error of that magnitude and apologetic of the consequences of their blunder. Not Doctor Death. She would not give even a pathetic, "Oops, my bad. I misread her chart. Sorry for turning your mother into an opioid zombie." No apologies from Doctor Death.

I told her the same complaints I had been telling the Hospice workers. I told her how Mom was overmedicated. I told her the constipation caused the worst of her suffering. How all her suffering had been caused by the drugs, not the cancer.

Doctor Death said, "Maybe we overmedicated your mother before, but we will not do that again. We will give her a small amount of Methadone to keep her baseline pain in check. We know the right dose now of Oxycodone, a half a pill for break through pain."

You know how she knew the right dose, not from any analysis, but from the one golden pill she gave my mother earlier. I said, "You are repeating the same mistakes you made before. Mom is going to get constipated. Her bowels will shut down. She will not eat. She will be in pain from the drugs."

Doctor Death said, "All opioids cause constipation but we will take care of that so she does not suffer. We will give her a laxative and enemas."

I told Doctor Death, Mom should never have been on those drugs. I told her that I almost had Mom off Lorazepam. Once off the Lorazepam, Mom would be drug free for the first time. We could see what was going on with Mom. We could tell if she was suffering from the cancer or the drugs. If Mom went on Methadone now, we would never give Mom a chance to be drug free. If we did things my way, that gave us the option of doing both. We could get Mom free of the drugs. We could find out what was going on. We could always give Mom more drugs later. There was no downside to doing things my way. My way kept all options open. My way afforded the best diagnosis. My way was the only way to identify what was hurting Mom.

Doctor Death insisted on putting Mom on Methadone now. She said, "Addiction does not matter. The important thing is to keep your mother comfortable."

Back to that, keeping comfortable? How can you be comfortable when your bowels do not work. We had a long fight. I said, "Only two weeks ago, Mom said she did not want to go on Methadone."

Doctor Death said, "What your mother said two weeks ago does not matter. She is no longer able to make her own decisions."

Typical. When Mom said what they wanted her to do, they said that was Mom's choice. When Mom did not say what they wanted her to do, they said Mom was not competent. We could have asked my mom right then, but Doctor Death had just given my mother Oxycodone and Mom was in a drugged haze.

Doctor Death insisted, "I am responsible for your mother's care. You do not have power of attorney over her healthcare. I am giving her Methadone." She said I could not stop her.

I said, "If I have no say so over the drugs Mom is getting, I want to be responsible for her nutrition. I want her to eat only the best foods. I want to control her diet."

Doctor Death said, "Nutrition does not matter."

Issues With Hospice

1. Their arrogance.

2. Not heeding warnings.

3. Putting my mother back on drugs once she was off them.

4. Depriving us of a chance to save my mother.

5. Repeating the same errors.

6. Giving my mother worse drugs.

Chapter 17 Alprazolam

מְכַלְכֵּל חַיִּים בְּחֶסֶד .

מְחַיֵּה מֵתִים בְּרַחֲמִים רַבִּים .

You sustain the living with loving kindness.
Revive the dead to life with great mercy.

~ Amidah, Jewish service central prayer

Alprazolam

Brand name Xanax. Drug class benzodiazepine. A sedative. Combining with other substances can slow breathing and possibly lead to death.

Can cause paranoia, impaired judgment, constipation, addiction, depressed mood, suicide thoughts, confusion, agitation, hallucinations, and severe breathing problems.

Abrupt discontinuation after prolonged use can lead to withdrawal symptoms. Patients should taper off slowly rather than abruptly stopping.

When Doctor Death put Mom on Methadone, she also switched Mom from Lorazepam to Alprazolam. The doctor said Alprazolam would be easier to taper off of. Alprazolam was longer lasting. The pill had a score that allowed you to cut the pill in half to give a smaller dose.

She was wrong. I probably could have stopped giving my mother Lorazepam then and there, but I had no experience. I was afraid to stop, even though her doses were small and far apart.

Doctor Death gave us a schedule for the Alprazolam, so much so often. After a week, I could see Mom was getting worse. I adjusted the spreadsheet I had made for Lorazepam to calculate the dose Mom was getting from Alprazolam based on that drug's half-life and potency. Even though we were giving Mom half the dose of Alprazolam that we had been giving her of Lorazepam, Alprazolam was twice as potent. Worse, the half-life of Alprazolam was double that of Lorazepam. That means more Alprazolam was in Mom's system longer. Comparing the numbers from Doctor Death's dosing schedule to where we had been with Mom's Lorazepam tapering, my mother had been set back three weeks.

I was so mad. I had not learned my lesson. The doctor had addicted my mother to Alprazolam. How many addictions was this for my mother, this 84 year-old woman who had had no drug addictions in her life? Let us count: Escitalopram, Oxycodone, Lorazepam, Oxycodone again, Alprazolam, and Methadone. Five by Hospice in a period of three months. Remember, this has not been to treat pain from cancer. This has been to treat pain caused by the drugs themselves.

My mother went through the agonies of withdrawal again now from the Alprazolam. Three weeks later, Janet said she talked to a psychiatrist at work, who said we could stop giving my mom the drug. That is what we did. Finally, nearly four months after going into the hospital, Mom was off the benzodiazepines, drugs she should never have been on in the first place.

You might ask at that point, why bother getting my mother off the drugs? She did not have long to live anyway. My sister asked that question too and answered the question herself. Every night, in my sister's words, my mother "was sun-downing". Mom was going berserk from the drug. Besides suffering from withdrawal symptoms at the end of her cycle, Mom was having an adverse reaction from getting the drug. She had to be taken off that drug.

Issues With Hospice

1. Giving my mother Alprazolam.

2. Ignorantly prescribing a drug without calculating dosage amounts.

3. Addicting my mother to yet another drug Alprazolam.

Chapter 18 Methadone

רְפָאֵנ וּ' וְנֵרָפֵא.

Heal us Hashem and we shall be healed

~ Amidah, Jewish service central prayer

Methadone

A narcotic. Can treat moderate to severe pain. Has a much longer duration of action than other opioids.

Side effects include sedation, alteration in cognitive and sensory efficiency, respiratory depression, nausea, vomiting, constipation, urinary retention, and concentration disorders.

Upon repeated administration, tolerance may develop. Can produce drug dependence. Withdrawal symptoms are similar to those of other opioids, but are less severe, slower in onset, and last longer.

Janet and I had terrible fights over my mother's medical treatment. These fights upset her family because they had never seen my sister like this. But I had. I am one year older than her and know her better than anyone.

In the movie "Good Will Hunting" Matt Damon's character has an emotional fight with his girlfriend Minnie Driver's character. He walks out on her. They do not talk to each other again. In the same movie, Robin Williams' character and

Professor Gerald Lambeau (Stellan Skarsgard) have terrible fights. They were former college roommates. Both are now professors. They insult each other, call each other names, make hard accusations, but they do not walk out on each other. They do not end their relationship.

During one family fight, my sister tried to walk out on my dad. He yelled at her, "Come back here and fight like a man. You cannot walk out on a fight." I have heard my sister say about her own family, they are all a bunch of wimps, no one will fight. Fighting is healthy. Fighting may be the only way to get people to express their deep seated emotions.

Whenever you have a relationship with someone, there are times when you will disagree on things that are important to you. You have to make up your mind that the important thing is to keep your relationship. You are going to win some. You are going to lose some. Whatever happens, the present will become the past. The past does not matter. The only thing that matters is keeping your relationship going forward.

Mom's Methadone schedule was one half pill early in the morning and one half pill in the evening. On the days Janet watched my mother, my sister gave my mother both her Methadone pills. On the days I watched my mother, I skipped giving my mother the morning pill. My sister still gave my mother the evening pill. While my sister had gone along with Doctor Death, my sister was not totally convinced.

Before taking any drug, go online and search for the name of the drug followed by the word "withdrawal", as in "methadone withdrawal". You will learn more, faster, about what you need to know than any other way. Methadone is a bad drug. Methadone is synthetic. Methadone saturates your body. Methadone is addictive. Methadone has a long half-life, staying in your system for five days. Due to the long half-life, Methadone is difficult to withdraw from. There are more deaths from Methadone than any other prescription drug. Deaths from Methadone are under reported. Methadone killed my mother, but my mother's death will be attributed to cancer, not Methadone. That is probably true of other prescription drugs too.

As soon as my mother went on Methadone, my mother's bowels shut down again. This time worse. She did not have another bowel movement on her own again. If you are on Oxycodone and only taking one pill a day, you could stop for a couple days. Your bowels start working again. Not so with Methadone. You have to wait five days for the Methadone to clear your system to get your bowels working. However, if you do not take Methadone every day, the withdrawals symptoms start right away. You have to suffer through five days of withdrawal before you can poop.

When Mom's bowels shut down, she was in constant pain. When asked where she hurt, Mom would move her hand across her midsection from one side to the other. Amy, remember Amy from dancing, used to work for Hospice and knew Doctor Death. Amy said that if the pain was under the ribs, the pain was from constipation in the bowels. I asked Mom if the pain was under her ribs. She said yes.

My plan of treating Mom with the most nutritious, anti-cancer diet and building up her immune system was subverted. Mom was barely eating. With her bowels shut down, what nutrition could she get anyway? People say that most of your immune system is in your bowels. I was shocked that Hospice thought nothing of intentionally shutting down my mother's digestive system.

Usually cancer does not kill you directly. Usually you die when your organs shut down. Cancer was not shutting down Mom's organs, not yet. Hospice was giving cancer a hand though. Hospice was intentionally shutting down Mom's bowels, you know, to keep Mom comfortable.

Hospice thought nothing of taking away my mother's mind either. Once again my mother, though not in a stupor, was confused. Much of what she said was nonsensical. My mother did not have dementia. The cause of her confusion was the Methadone. Surely not having a functional digestive system contributed to her erratic mental condition.

Mom was still able to get out of bed and onto the toilet or into the wheelchair. We could take her out of the room. At this point Mom was no longer suffering from Alprazolam. Mom had two pains. One was the pain in her right hip, caused by her fall. Mom did not need Methadone for a bruise. Mom's other pain was the severe, constant pain in her bowels. Doctor Death had instructed us to give my mother half an Oxycodone for break through pain. Oxycodone also causes constipation. When my mother complained more than normal, my sisters gave my mother half an Oxycodone which was usually once a day. Bizarrely, Hospice was giving my mother Methadone and Oxycodone to treat the pain caused by the constipation the Methadone and Oxycodone induced.

Everything happened like I told Hospice it would. You might say Hospice made the same mistake again. I do not think so. If I could predict correctly with my experience limited to this one patient, Doctor Death, with her vast experience, knew well what was going to happen. Doctor Death said Mom would be dead in three weeks. I believe Doctor Death knew the drugs would kill my mother. Remember Doctor Death did not change her prognosis when she found out she read my mother's chart wrong and that my mother did not have cancer throughout her body.

After the first two weeks, I had hopes that Mom may not have become overly addicted to the Methadone. I thought we might be able to get her off the Methadone without her suffering from too severe withdrawal symptoms. I badgered Janet to get Mom off the Methadone while we still had a chance. Methadone was obviously killing my mother. Mom was barely eating. All her pains were caused by the Methadone. My sister went along with my tapering Mom off the Methadone. Getting Mom off Methadone was not easy. Instead of tapering, we should have stopped altogether and fired Hospice.

Three weeks into the Methadone the pain in my Mom's left hip and middle back reappeared where her tumors had been. I thought this was strange. I wondered if Methadone caused the tumors to grow, either directly by some mechanism enhancing tumor growth, or by inhibiting the immune system, or by preventing good nutrition. Turns out by all three.

Four weeks into the Methadone, Doctor Death came by of her own accord. She met with Mom. Doctor Death said to my mother, "I am surprised to see you are still here."

My mother asked, "Where did you expect me to be?"

"In Heaven," answered Doctor Death in a gentle voice.

Whatever the tone, I was horrified by the insensitivity. Mom was not ready to die. What Mom wanted was the pain to stop. Some people are ready to die. Our neighbor Tex Lindgren was 97 years old. He was Swedish. He was strong like a Viking. He fell and his wife Joan called me to help pick him up. He was so muscular, I could barely get him off the ground. For the last two years, he had a catheter. He did not like being old. He was ready to die. You could say something like, "In Heaven," to him, although he did not believe in Heaven.

I told Doctor Death the worst pains my mother was suffering from were caused by the constipation. Mom indicated the pain hurt all across her midsection. Mom swept her hand from one side to the other to show where she hurt, right where her bowels were. Right where you would move your hand to show where you were having gas pains.

Doctor Death put her stethoscope on the same spot. She listened for three seconds, no joke and no exaggeration. Doctor Death said, "I hear normal sounds. Her bowels are not obstructed. The pain is not caused by constipation."

Really, a three second diagnosis has determined the pain cannot be from her bowels? She had not had a bowel movement on her own in a month.

I asked, "Why is there pain all across her bowels from one side to the other?"

Doctor Death said, "The pain is probably radiating from her hip."

I said, "The pain is radiating from her hip all the way up into her bowels without causing pain in between? Why is there pain on her right side?"

Doctor Death said, "The pain is probably radiating from her right hip."

I said, "The pain in her right hip is from when she fell." I asked, "Why is there pain under her ribs?"

Doctor Death said, "That pain is probably radiating from the tumor in her back."

I said, "The tumor in her back is radiating pain around to her front to exactly where her bowels are? And without causing pain in the intervening area? This all seems unlikely."

Occam's Razor, the simplest explanation was the pain was coming from Mom's bowels caused by the Methadone.

Doctor Death said, "We have already established the pain is not from her bowels, so the pain must be from the cancer."

Doctor Death's explanation was nonsense, but she was not saying that for my benefit. Doctor Death was saying that for my sister's benefit to give my sister some reason to hang on to. Imagine if Doctor Death admitted the pain was caused by the Methadone.

I asked about trying medical marijuana. I told Doctor Death my sister's best friend Debbie, a cardiologist in Tampa, was prescribing marijuana for appetite for her patients. There were many reports online about pain relief using marijuana. Marijuana reputedly had anti-cancer benefits as well, supposedly inhibiting tumor growth. If marijuana worked for my mother, the benefits could be working bowels, increased appetite, mood enhancement, inhibited tumor growth, and pain relief.

Doctor Death refused to consider marijuana, saying, "Marijuana does not relieve pain."

Doctor Death was not happy I was weaning Mom off Methadone. We had another big fight. Doctor Death threatened me, "If you do not give her the Methadone, I will bar you from the premises."

I said, "I am not going to give my mother Methadone."

They decided Janet would give Mom the Methadone.

A few days later the nurse called Janet. The nurse threatened to call Social Services to take Mom away if we did not give Mom the Methadone.

We tried to find something to relieve Mom's pain from constipation, which was agonizing her. My cousin Bill, the gastroenterologist, suggested Movantik. My good friend Philip Schwartz, whose mother Libby passed away recently at 91 from ovarian cancer, found an article that listed the University of Chicago Medical Center as the source. The article was about a chemist whose friend was dying of cancer. His friend was suffering from opioid induced constipation. The chemist invented a drug that blocked the action of opioids in the body, but the molecule was too big to pass the blood brain barrier so the opioids still worked to relieve pain in the brain. People given that drug lived longer. Their tumor growth slowed, in some cases tumors shrunk. People had already suspected opioids induced tumor growth before then. Now there was proof. I was right. Opioids cause cancer tumors to grow faster.

Methadone is the worst. My friend June said, "I would not give Methadone to my worst enemy." June was looking after her parents who were renowned, healthcare scientists living into their 90s. With Oxycodone, at least the drug leaves your system after six hours. Methadone works by saturating your body so the tumors always have a supply of opioids to promote their growth. You put someone with cancer on Methadone, they are a dead man.

I am going to rush through this part, because I do not want to dwell on my mother's suffering which was horrible.

Mom's hip and back got worse. Mom could no longer get out of bed to get on the toilet. Mom could barely move around in bed. Mom quickly developed two large, stage 2 bed sores, one on her coccyx and one in the middle of her back. Bed sores are difficult to heal. Bed sores can kill you. Let me caution you. Bed sores can appear before you know what is happening. If you are caring for someone who is bedridden, you must be vigilant in protecting against bed sores. I ordered a medical air mattress to treat Mom's bed sores, but the mattress arrived too late to do any good. If you are caring for someone who is bedridden, I would get the air mattress right away. I do not know if they work, but without one, we had a disaster.

Mom's left ribs hurt her. This was a new pain. Hospice blamed this new pain on the cancer. I believe this was a pulled muscle caused by the Hospice healthcare worker roughing Mom up while bathing Mom. Mom was now almost dead weight and hard to move. Nothing against the healthcare worker. That can happen. The pain was treated with a lidocaine patch, which was effective. Eventually the rib pain went away, so not cancer.

The pain in Mom's right hip had gone away, so not cancer. Mom now had six pains: (1) constipation, (2) coccyx bed sore, (3) back bed sore, (4) left hip tumor, (5) back tumor, and (6) left ribs. I attribute all six pains directly or indirectly to the Methadone. I believe the Methadone caused the tumors to come back. The tumors left Mom bedridden and mostly stuck in one position. Being stuck in one position in bed caused the bed sores. Mom's inability to move caused the healthcare worker to strain Mom's ribs. If Mom had not been on Methadone, I do not think she would have had any of these pains at this time.

Sure, if the tumors came back some time in the future, these pains would be directly attributable to the cancer. However, if she was not on Methadone, and she was eating healthy, maybe the tumors would not have come back for years, or maybe not at all. Remember my friend's mother, who had lung cancer, lived to die of something else.

Mom lived another six weeks. Much of the time she slept. She did not leave the room because she could not get into the wheelchair. One day she mumbled, "Can I get out of this room like a person." I tried unsuccessfully to find a mobile recliner. Every day was worse than the one before. No need for you to know more details.

The last week or two Mom had severe problems breathing. Her heart was racing continuously around 120 beats per minute. Mom had an oxygen tube blowing into her nose but was breathing through her mouth. I moved the tube to her mouth. Her breathing calmed down. Her heart slowed to a more normal 80 beats per minute. At the same time, Tex Lindgren went into the hospital because of complications with the catheter. From the hospital he went to Hospice. I blamed the Methadone for Mom's breathing problems. Breathing problems are a side effect of opioids. As noted in the chapter on Oxycodone, "Oxycodone is more likely to cause breathing problems in older adults and people who are severely ill, malnourished, or otherwise debilitated." All true of my mother. Of course, Mom did have lung cancer. Opioids do cause the tumors to grow faster. Her breathing problems could have been caused by the tumors in her lungs. However, I suspect the opioids for yet another reason.

Issues With Hospice

1. Giving my mother Methadone.

2. Not giving my mother a chance to get better.

3. Taking away my mother's mind a second time.

4. Shutting down my mother's digestive system intentionally.

5. Inducing my mother's tumors to grow faster.

6. Causing my mother to develop severe bed sores.

7. The misery they put my mother through.

Chapter 19 Morphine

שֶׁוּ רַחֵם עָלֵינוּ וְתִמְחָל לָנוּ עַל כָּל חַטֹּאתֵינ .

Have compassion on us and forgive us for all our sins.

~ Jewish prayer

Morphine

An opioid. Similar to natural pain killers made in our body called endorphins. Opioids block pain signals from traveling along the nerves to the brain.

From: The adverse effects of morphine ... for chronic cancer pain - Paul Glare 1, ... PMID: 17060284

Little information is available about morphine side effects for chronic cancer pain although it has been widely used for more than 30 years. Dry mouth was the most common (95%); Sedation and constipation were frequent (88%). Although constipation, nausea, and sedation are well described as side effects, others such as dry mouth appear to be underestimated. Validated measures are needed.

Hospice left us with Morphine to give to my mother on a schedule, plus more as needed. Hospice was finally in their element now that Mom was clearly dying. They gave us a booklet explaining what happened at end of life. They told us what to expect. They said it is normal for the patient to extend their neck, turning their face upward to gasp for breath. They said this and other behaviors were signs the body was preparing to die.

What they said did not make sense to me. What this looked like was Mom was dying from what I will call opioid poisoning. That the Hospice workers were so familiar with this process, that they even had a booklet outlining the process, makes me think they are killing many people with opioid poisoning. Hospice treats people dying of all sorts of things, not only lung cancer. You can accept that a lung cancer patient may have trouble breathing, but everyone? Hospice is probably loading many people up on Oxycodone, Methadone, Morphine, and any other number of opioid drugs. That is why, I suspect, they all go through a predictable, dying process. They are all dying of opioid poisoning.

What do I mean by opioid poisoning? Opioid poisoning is a series of insults to the body caused by opioids. These insults compound health problems until the person stops drinking. These health problems include shutting down of the digestive system, malnutrition, weakening of the immune system, disruption of the mind, depression of other bodily functions such as breathing, lack of exercise, loss of muscle, being bedridden, bed sores, infections, loss of appetite, starvation and so on. The final one, the one they can no longer survive, is when they stop drinking. In my mother's case, she stopped drinking because she could no longer swallow. I suspect the cause of death is when their heart stops from dehydration.

Mom stopped eating and drinking on Wednesday July 13. The last four days were torture. She was gasping for breath.

She was dying from lack of water, I presume. A terrible way to go.

If you give someone too much Morphine, they stop breathing. Euthanasia is illegal in Florida. Accidentally overdosing someone on Morphine is not illegal. Janet asked me if I wanted to give Mom extra morphine. Killing Mom would have been merciful, but I could not bring myself to kill my mother. I told my sister, she could. She did not either. Letting my mother suffer for four days is one thing that haunts me.

Sometime afterwards, I ran into a friend Michelle, who had gone through similar medical issues with her mother and brother. Michelle told me that morphine can cause people to have trouble breathing and can prevent people from swallowing. Searching online, I corroborated these effects of morphine.

I now believe my mother's breathing problems were a direct result of the morphine, not the cancer. Worse, I believe the morphine, not the cancer, was preventing her from swallowing. Her inability to swallow was the cause of her death because she could no longer drink.

Issues With Hospice

1. Poisoning my mother with opioids.

2. Making my mother die from lack of water.

3. Killing my mother, who I believe would be alive as I write this.

Chapter 20 Living Your Life

אֱלֹהַ . נְשָׁמָה שֶׁ נָּתַתָּ בִּי טְהוֹרָה הִיא .

אַתָּה בְרָאתָו . אַתָּה יְצַרְתָּו . אַתָּה נְפַחְתָּה בּ .

וְאַתָּה מְשַׁמְּרָה בְּקִרְבּ .

וְאַתָּה עָתִיד לִטְּלָה מִמֶּנִּ . וּלְהַחֲזִירָה בִּי לֶעָתִיד לָבוֹא .

כָּל זְמַן שֶׁהַנְּשָׁמָה בְּקִרְבִּי מוֹדֶה אֲנִי לְנָ נֶיךְ

ו ' אֱלֹהַי וֵאלֹהֵי אֲבוֹת . רִבּוֹן כָּל הַמַּעֲשִׂים אֲדוֹן כָּל

הַנְּשָׁמוֹו :

בָּרוּךְ אַתָּו ו ' הַמַּחֲזִיר נְשָׁמוֹת לִפְגָרִים מֵתִינ :

My God, the soul you have given me is pure. You
created it. You formed it. You blew it into me.
And you preserve it within me. And you will
take it from me, and restore it to me in the
hereafter.
As long as my soul is within me, I give thanks
before You, Hashem my God and God of my
fathers, Master of all creation, Lord of all souls.
Blessed are You Hashem, Who restores souls to
the dead.

~ Elohai Neshama, My God, the Soul, Jewish
blessing

The last moments, Mom stopped gasping for air.

Janet and I held Mom's hands. She breathed peacefully for
a couple of minutes. Mom's heart stopped. We said, "Shema
Yisrael, Adonai Eloheinu, Adonai Echad".

Tex Lindgren passed away two hours after Mom. They lived across the street from each other for 45 years. Mom's longtime friends Freda Green, Arlene Greer, and Regina Plutzky passed away over the next few months. I remember my dad looking through old family photo albums pointing at people, saying, "Dead, dead, dead."

After I spoke at the synagogue during Mom's ceremony, Rabbi Kaiman spoke. Thirteen years earlier the Rabbi spoke at my father's passing. The Rabbi had just started at our synagogue then. The Rabbi did not know my father. The Rabbi knew my mother well. He told funny stories about Mom and her friends that I did not know.

We went to the synagogue's cemetery. There was a short ceremony. I put the first shovel full of dirt on my mother's grave with the shovel blade upside down. I put a stone on my dad's headstone. The congregation formed a line on either side as we walked out. We rinsed our hands upon leaving.

We went back to my house to sit Shiva. The congregation came over. The ladies made sure Janet, Randi, and I ate first. The community came by every day. They brought our meals. We felt like we had fifty mothers.

After Shiva, at the store, I ran into Mom's friend Roz Shever. Roz said to me, "It is time to get back living your life."

Two weeks later Janis Tillman knocked on my door. She asked if Mom wanted the garden weeded again. I told her Mom passed away three weeks ago.

"Oh no, not your mom," Janis said. "She was so vigorous. I just saw her a few months ago. She was walking around the neighborhood. She stopped to talk with me. She was chatty. 'Here I go, another lap,' she said."

We talked. Her mom had passed away recently too.

"There is nothing like when your momma goes. It is going to be difficult. If you had a good momma, one that was kind, that loved you. I know your momma was like that. You have to pray. You have to cry. Read Psalm 91. The Lord created the universe. He can get you through this. I know this is hard on you."

I told her Mom would still be alive, but Hospice killed Mom with all the drugs.

Janis said, "I know that is what they do. They tried to drug my momma, but we took her off those drugs."

I told her I started taking care of the yard since Mom passed. I told her I felt bad that I did not garden when Mom was alive.

Janis said, "I talk to my momma every day. I cry. Everyone feels bad. Momma I wish I did this and momma I wish I did that. All you can do is go forward. That is what your momma would want."

When I was seventeen years old, I realized I was going to die one day. I was scared. I went into my mother's room. I told her what I was thinking.

The only relative that had passed away in my life till then was my Grandma Ida's brother Willy. My mother said something that comforted me for the time being. Mom said, "When I die, I think I will be with Uncle Willy and all the other people we love."

* * *

The End

Epilogue

יְבָרֶכְךָ וֹ' וְיִשְׁמְרֶךָ׃

יָאֵו וֹ' פָּנָיו אֵלֶיךָ וִיחֻנֶּךָּ׃

יִשָּׂא וֹ' פָּנָיו אֵלֶיךָ וְיָשֵׂם לְךָ שָׁלוֹם׃

May Hashem bless you and guard you.
May Hashem shine His face upon you and treat
you graciously.
May Hashem lift His face towards you and grant
you peace.

~ Blessing of the Kohanim, Priests

Six Years Later in 2022

Lawsuits

Three years after my mother's passing, Soojin and I were on a bus tour in Argentina to see Aconcagua, the highest mountain in the Americas. We were the only ones that spoke English, not even the tour guide, except for a huge young man from California. We befriended him.

His name was Ian. He was 27 years old, six feet five inches tall, weighed over 300 pounds, and was a former football player. He was traveling around South America alone until his girlfriend could join him.

That I wrote this book came out in conversation. Ian had a lot to say. Ian's mother was a doctor. She retired recently frustrated over the same complaints I had about healthcare. Ian worked for a law firm that was suing hospices in California for the kind of medical practices that happened to us. He said the hospice behaviors I was complaining about were common. When I got home, I looked up hospice lawsuits in California. There were many results.

Opioids and Benzodiazepines

There is an opioid crisis in the United States that has worsened. The manufacturer of Oxycontin was sued in West Virginia. The judge, agreeing with me, blamed the doctors for prescribing the medication, not the manufacturer. The Veterans Administration, where my sister works, no longer prescribes opioids or benzodiazepines.

Covid

Morris Sternberger died in 2020 at the age of 91 from Covid. He lived with his brother-in-law Marvin Goldstein. Marvin died at the age of 96 from Covid at the same time. Stanley Brownstein, my brother-in-law Steve's father, died at the age of 91 from Covid in 2020. Soojin's cousin Bomi, who we had visited in Brazil two weeks before meeting Ian, died at the age of 39 from Covid in 2022. All had their appropriate vaccines.

Family

Morris' sister Laura is currently a healthy 91. I had lunch yesterday with my nephew Josh who is visiting. My sister Randi moved in with me to go to graduate school at the University of Florida. She got her master's degree. UF immediately hired her. We share an office. She is sitting behind me as I write this. Randi, my other sister Janet, and my brother-in-law Steve, and I have Shabbat dinner together most Friday nights.

Afterward Notes

צוֹפֶה וְיוֹדֵעַ סְתָרֵינוּ , מַבִּיט לְסוֹף דָּבָר בְּקַדְמָת .

He watches and knows our secrets, seeing the end of something at its beginning.

~ Yigdal, Jewish liturgical song

I have tried to keep the narrative of the story of my mother's illness moving along. That story was how Hospice killed my mother through drug misuse. The story line mostly followed what happened.

The story raises many questions such as how could such a thing happen? To avoid bogging down the story with speculations to this question, and others, as well as to provide other information related to the story, I have included this section of notes.

A1 Why I Wrote This Book

יִהְיוּ לְרָצוֹן אִמְרֵי פִי וְהֶגְיוֹן לִבִּי לְפָנֶיךָ וּ ' צוּרִי וְגוֹאֲלִ :

May the words of my mouth and the meditation of my heart be acceptable to You, Hashem my Rock and my Redeemer.

~ Amidah, Jewish service central prayer

When I started at IBM in 1981, I worked in a large operations room with more than a dozen people. On the other side of the room were some computer operators that smoked. I complained to management about the smoke. IBM had an open door policy. This meant you could complain up the management chain as high as you liked. I went to the highest levels of management in my division. I was sent to the head of Human Resources. He was a pipe smoker. He said, "Are there large clumps of smoke floating around the room?" I lost that battle.

Soon we moved out of the operations room into our own offices. Non-smokers were put with non-smokers and smokers with smokers, possibly from my efforts. There was still smoke in the air, but not as bad. Though I was right, I gave up the fight. There were other people elsewhere that did not give up the fight. Within a few years all of IBM campuses were smoke free. Today, most of the public spaces in the United States are smoke free.

When my mother was diagnosed with cancer, my plan was to give Mom the best nutrition. Put her on an anti-cancer diet. Exercise her. Keep her mind alert. Encourage her to see friends. Help her to feel as good as possible. Use the oncologist and the radiation oncologist for the kind of care my mother wanted. If she did not want aggressive chemotherapy and surgery, there were still good options that were not traumatizing. This was the best plan for my mother. I had never heard the term palliative care.

Hospice subverted my plan by pretending to be something they are not. My purpose in this book is to show how Hospice relentlessly pursued their mission of moving people through the system. Regardless of what is best for the patient, regardless of the evidence put in front of them, Hospice would not change course.

At one time, Hospice was only for the dying, those people who had days to live with no other options. Hospice methods may be acceptable for those people. Hospice has expanded their service to include people who want palliative care, whose time left is unknown, like my mother. Hospice is pushing themselves onto people as palliative care specialists. They are not.

Caring for people whose life expectancy is unknown requires a different approach than for those already stepping through death's door. Yet Hospice has not changed their practices. Hospice applies the same methods to those people who are, or could be, still living their life as to those about to die. That is wrong, with torturous consequences, as what happened to my mother. To keep this point clear, this book has mostly limited the story to the misbehavior of Hospice.

I wrote this book in part so you could judge for yourself: was Hospice providing palliative care or was Hospice doing what Hospice always does, end-of-life care. See the section in these notes titled "Palliative Care Verses Hospice Care" taken from the National Institute for Health to see what palliative care is supposed to be. Here are selected notes from that page.

"Palliative care is care given to improve the quality of life of patients who have a serious or life-threatening disease, such as cancer. The goal of palliative care is to prevent or treat, as early as possible, the symptoms and side effects of the disease and its treatment".

"The goal is to maintain the best possible quality of life."

"Often, palliative care specialists work as part of a multidisciplinary team to coordinate care. This palliative care team may consist of ... registered dieticians ... psychologists".

"Palliative care is given in addition to cancer treatment."

"Although hospice care has the same principles of comfort and support, palliative care is offered earlier in the disease process. As noted above, a person's cancer treatment continues to be administered and assessed while he or she is receiving palliative care."

What Hospice told my mother was one thing. What they actually did had nothing to do with palliative care. All Hospice did was drug my mother until she died. My objection is not incompetence. I would not have written this book if Hospice was simply incompetent. The people working for Hospice knew what they were doing. My objection is intention. Hospice had no intention of providing palliative care. Had Hospice changed course when I informed them of their mistreatment of my mother, they would only have been incompetent in the beginning which is forgivable. What Hospice did when I informed them of their mistreatment was argue with me. When that did not work, they threatened to bar me from the premises and call Social Services to remove my mother. That is intention.

Let us take a look back at Hospice's intention. Hospice's plan was nutrition does not matter, addiction does not matter. Hospice plan was to drug my mother until she died, regardless of consequences. The drugs shut down her bowels, suppressed her appetite, prevented her from getting nutrition, suppressed her immune system, induced her cancer tumors to grow, kept her bedridden, caused bed sores, caused her to lose her muscle strength, and caused her to lose her mind. When I informed Hospice of their behavior, they gave my mother worse drugs and sought to get rid of me.

Why did Hospice do what they did? We can speculate. The Hospice organization seeks to grow more powerful, as so many organizations do. Hospice expands their services into palliative care to do so. Hospice motivates their sales people to get palliative patients, which they do. Hospice fails to institute palliative care services. Instead Hospice applies their end-of-life services to their palliative care patients. The result is the terrible months my mother suffered.

How to solve the problem? The right way to solve the Hospice problem is for Hospice to stick with what they know, end-of-life care and be satisfied with their size. Hospice does not need to grow bigger. The wrong way is for Hospice to try to acquire palliative care expertise which is a conflict in objective. As demonstrated by Doctor Death, one doctor cannot be both an end-of-life specialist and a palliative care specialist. The goals are different.

I wrote this book during my mourning process because I had something to say. Like any book, there are multiple themes. Like any theme, the complaint lodged against Hospice picks at larger, underlying issues in our society. Before getting on with my life, I wanted to attempt to contribute to the battle to choose life.

A2 Lashon Hara - Evil Speech

Take a feather pillow, cut it open, and scatter the feathers to the winds. Now, go and gather the feathers. Because you can no more make amends for the damage your words have done than you can recollect the feathers.

~ Jewish tale

I have avoided naming names for I do not seek to harm individuals. While I opposed their intentions, all those involved in my mother's care, I believe, felt their intentions were best for Mom's welfare.

I did not want to go to medical school because I did not want to be around sick people all day long. That did not sound like much fun. Thankfully there are those who devote themselves to the care of those at the end-of-life. I am writing about the Hospice workers. They are doing holy work. They should be praised for their choice of profession.

I include Doctor Death, a person who should be appreciated for her choice of providing end-of-life care. She took the trouble to make two house calls to see my mother. She argued with me until I stopped arguing. She did not end the argument. She had the patience to wait me out. An impressive feat and compassionate one.

Jewish law forbids Lashon Hara, evil speech, which is derogatory speech about individuals, even if true. Jewish law requires you to reveal information to protect a person from immediate, serious harm. You are also permitted to reveal information if someone is entering into a relationship that he would not enter if he knew certain information.

A3 Jewish Mourning

I will always remember her generosity and hospitality when we came to visit.

~ Annie Berman, niece

Judaism is concerned with the living. Jewish prayer does include reference to life after death. The second blessing in the Amidah, the central Jewish prayer in the daily services, is "Blessed are You Hashem, Who revives the dead." Jews recite this three times a day, four times on Shabbat and holidays. Still mainstream Judaism is not much interested in what happens after you die. The Jewish mourning practices fulfill our obligation to the dead and provide a process for returning to live your life.

When we moved from New York to Florida, I never saw my friends from the old neighborhood again. When someone moves away, in a way, to you they may die. You may never speak to them again, but you may. Unlike dying, there is not finality. When you bury someone, you will not see them again in your lifetime. The act of putting someone in the ground is a finality. Your obligation to the dead ends when you bury them. It is then time to start the process of getting on with your life.

Technically, Jews mourn for seven people, mother, father, sister, brother, son, daughter, and spouse. Shiva is the first seven days. You stay at home. The last day you walk around the neighborhood symbolizing your return to the normal world. After Shiva, you return to work and most of your normal activities.

Shloshim is the first thirty days. You continue some mourning practices, such as saying the Kaddish blessing at synagogue and not cutting your hair, which explains the author's picture on the cover. You do not go to parties or public celebrations out of respect for the memory of those who passed. For people to see you out celebrating would be unseemly, "Yeay! I got the inheritance. Finally, the old codger died."

For all but your parents, your mourning period ends at the end of Shloshim. You mourn your parents for one year. There is a custom that after you die your soul spends the next twelve months reflecting on your life before joining the Holy One, blessed be He. Those that lived righteously join the Holy One one month early. Each time you say Kaddish for someone you help uplift the soul on the soul's journey. We stop saying Kaddish for our parent after eleven months because if we say Kaddish after the eleventh month, that would mean we did not believe our parent lived righteously.

After the mourning period, we say Kaddish on the anniversary of their death and during the Yitzkor Service during four holidays throughout the year. The Kaddish is an affirmation of life and has no mention of death.

A4 Faith

קָרוֹג וֹ ' לְכָל קֹרְאָיו

Near is Hashem to all who call Him

~ Psalm 145

As I prayed, "Master of the Universe, You created the universe, all things are possible to You, cure my mother of cancer." I wondered, why am I praying? If God is going to cure my mother of cancer, why let her get cancer in the first place?

I am a religious person. I do some of the things I am supposed to do. I go to synagogue regularly. I keep kosher, kind of. I keep Shabbat, kind of. I am not superstitious. I do not want to be foolish. There are two questions to answer. Is religion stupid? Is faith in God stupid?

The first question is simple to answer. Religion is not stupid. Faith in our tradition is easy for me. I love our tradition. This book gives you a glimpse how enriching life can be with religion. One rule of life is we rarely know what we missed. My friend Howard Cohen, an astronomy professor, says that seeing a total solar eclipse is the most spectacular natural event you will see in your lifetime. One that you will never forget. Yet, he says, there are people that would not go outside to see an eclipse passing over their head. They go on living their life oblivious to what they missed. We all do. Religion makes sense whether God exists or not. If you have a tradition you want to share with others, including those living before and after you, you have a religion. Religion, done in a way that works for you, is like living your life in color. Living your life without religion, is like living in black and white. You miss out on many enriching experiences. In this sense, you could say religion is culture.

The answer to the second question, is faith in God stupid, is not yet. Faith in what I believe is the Jewish conception of God is not stupid. No one has proven this conception of God to be false. Existence makes no sense. Free will makes no sense. Maybe one day someone will be able to explain these without God. For now, faith in God is still reasonable.

I saw Adin Steinsaltz, the Talmudic scholar, author of the Steinsaltz Talmud, friend of the Lubavitcher Rebbe, speak at the Boca Raton Synagogue. With his long white beard, he looked one hundred years old, although he was probably only sixty.

Someone asked him a question, beginning with, "Rabbi Steinsaltz".

Adin Steinsaltz interrupted, "I am not a rabbi."

During his talk, Adin Steinsaltz said, "faith was the hardest thing for me to come by."

Faith is hard for me too. At least the faith that God exists. I believe in God, kind of. I believe because believing the contrary, that God does not exist, requires faith too. I believe because I want to believe.

A5 Cards from Friends

כִּי מַלְאָכָיו יְצַוֶּה־לָּ֑ךְ לִֽשְׁמָרְךָ֗ בְּכָל־דְּרָכֶֽיךָ׃

He will command His angels to guard you wherever you go.

~ Psalm 91

My mother was living her life. Every day she went out with friends, the lunch bunch, the book club, the knitting circle; she went to movies, lectures and the theatre. She was busy. One day she went to lunch. The next day she went into the hospital.

What should have happened was she should have went on with her life, only now with cancer. Instead, her life ended that day, for her friends and for her. Between the hospital and hospice, she was on so many drugs, she was never able to function normally again.

My mother got many notes, frequently, maybe daily. Here is a sample. They are writing to my mother the way they knew her. The striking impression is they think they are writing to a cognizant person. My mother though was in a stupor. My mother was so drugged, she was unable to read or reply to any notes, or even comprehend them when my sister read the notes to my mother. The crime was my mother and her friends were deprived of any contact from the day my mother was diagnosed.

Hi Sweetie Edie,

Just wanting to say hello and to let you know you are in my thoughts.

Josh came by yesterday as he is going to stay with Prince next weekend and he looked like he had grown a foot since the last time we saw him.

My grandson graduated UF two weeks ago and is going to the D.C. area like Josh. Ben does not have a job, but his girlfriend is in the Navy for the next 5 years as she was at UF on a ROTC scholarship. He will look when he is there.

Love,
Roz

* * *

Dearest Edie,

I hope the spunky old broad on this card brings a smile to your face.

Like all of your friends, I am greatly saddened by your illness and hope you are comfortable and without pain.

In honor of your upcoming birthday I propose a toast to all the movies seen, to all the ribs consumed, and to all the laughs and good times shared.

I miss you my Brooklyn friend, and I send you much love, Myra

* * *

Dear Edie,

I hear you have a bird feeder right outside your window. The question is do you have any birds that are hanging around and maybe even singing you a song.

Tis a rainy day today and you cannot imagine how many times I have to wipe my Pumpkin's feet and mine too. I use my walker when I go out with Pumpkin just because it is easier to walk, but I have to clean up my foyer many, many times. Sometimes to go in through the garage, but then I have to be aware that the cat (who only thinks she belongs to me) does not get closed in the garage. And on and on and on. ...

Miss You, Carol

P.S. Hope I get a smile out of you

* * *

Feb 9, 2016

Dear Edie,

My heart hurts for you. It also hurts for me!

I think about you every day and wonder why I did not notice anything was wrong when we had our Ballyhoo lunch. You looked like the "fashionista" I always expect with your beautiful red jacket. Little did I know.

Since I cannot talk to you, I am going to send you some of the great memories I have with you and Shellie.

#1. How about the time we drove to Jacksonville with Randi and Karyn? Coming home we almost went to Georgia before we noticed!

#2 will be on the next card.

I love you and my life has been so much more exciting having known you and Shelly.

Thank You,
Diane

A6 Opioids Accelerate Tumor Growth

Methyl naltrexone was developed in 1979, so there has been evidence for a long time that opioids induced tumor growth. People may have suspected opioids accelerated tumor growth way before that. After all, I guessed that opioids caused tumors to grow faster in my one experience. People in the business must have been seeing this over and over again, from the beginning of opioid use in cancer patients. You would think that every doctor that prescribes opioids to cancer patients would know and warn their patients that opioid medication causes tumors to grow faster.

If you search for "Opioids Tumor Growth" and "Methadone Tumor Growth", you can find research indicating opioids promote tumor growth. You can also find research indicating Methadone can enhance the effect of cancer killing drugs in vitro. At least some tumor cells have many more opioid receptors than normal cells. Seemingly, depending on conditions, opioids can cause tumors to grow faster or can help drugs cause cancer cells to die. In my mother's case, Methadone appeared to cause her tumors to grow faster.

Here is one article from the United States government, medical research, publication website.

Treatment with methyl naltrexone is associated with increased survival in patients with advanced cancer. Ann Oncol. 2016 Nov;27(11):2032-2038. Epub 2016 Aug 29. Janku F1, Johnson LK2, Karp DD1, Atkins JT1, Singleton PA3,4, Moss J5.

Here are links to two articles on this topic on the University of Chicago hospitals website, as of October 9, 2017.

Common pain relief medication may encourage cancer growth. From November 18, 2009. ... a growing body of evidence is showing that opiate-based painkillers can stimulate the growth and spread of cancer cells. ...

http://www.uchospitals.edu/news/2009/20091119-pain-med.html

Evidence mounts for link between opioids and cancer growth. From March 21, 2012. Opioid drugs used to relieve pain in postoperative and chronic cancer patients may stimulate the growth and spread of tumors ...

http://www.uchospitals.edu/news/2012/20120321-opioid.html

A7 Research Studies

בָּרוּךְ אַתָּה ו ' אֱלֹהֵינוּ מֶלֶךְ הָעוֹלָם . אֲשֶׁר נָתַן לַשֶּׂכְוִי בִינָה
לְהַבְחִין בֵּין יוֹם וּבֵין לָיְלָה .

Blessed are You Hashem our God, King of the Universe, Who gave the rooster insight to distinguish between day and night.

~ Jewish morning blessing upon hearing the cock crow

The first section I have labeled Cancer Inhibitors, for research on various natural substances that fight cancer. I searched for studies on lung cancer with natural substances. I listed the ones that popped up first. This is a miniscule sample. There are thousands of papers on many individual substances alone.

The second section I have labeled Cancer Promoters for research findings that promote cancer growth. Some of the studies that popped up in my first search were about non-natural substances that promoted cancer. I listed a small number of those in the second section to contrast with the natural substances.

Suppose my mother's cancer fell into the 25% of slow growing cancer cases as in this study.

Estimating over diagnosis in low-dose computed tomography screening for lung cancer: a cohort study. Ann Intern Med. 2012 Dec 4 ;157(11):776-84. PMID: 23208167

Conclusion: Slow-growing or indolent cancer comprised approximately 25% of incident cases, many of which may have been over diagnosed. To limit overtreatment in these cases, minimally invasive limited resection and nonsurgical treatments should be investigated.

This raises the question as to why some cancers are slow growing. Perhaps cancer grows slower in bodies that are more inhospitable to cancer and faster in bodies that have a more favorable environment for cancer growth. What would determine how hospitable your body is to cancer? What you eat, drink, breath, do. What drugs you take. What therapies you under go.

This study reports on a case similar to my mother's, successfully using herbal medicine.

Rapid bone repair in a patient with lung cancer metastases to the spine using a novel herbal medicine: A case report. Rong Pu, Qianhong Zhao, Zhimei Li, Lingyan Zhang, Xiaolu Luo, Yangji Zeren, Cui Yu, and Xianyong Li1. Oncol Lett. 2016 Sep; 12(3): 2023–2027. Published online 2016 Jul 18. doi: 10.3892/ol.2016.4879. PMCID: PMC4998527. PMID: 27602132

In conclusion, the present study describes a case in which herbal medicine promoted tumor regression and bone repair, with an improved quality of life in a short period of time. It is unclear whether the combination of herbal medicine and bisphosphonates synergistically enhanced bone repair. The study demonstrated a novel individualized approach to treat lung cancer patients ...

Afterward Notes

Once the tumors in my mother's hip and back were shrunk from the radiation, suppose she was on an anti-cancer diet, avoiding cancer promoters and off drugs; in particular off opioids that have been shown to promote tumor growth. Could she have gone back to living her life? Would the tumors have grown? How quickly? Maybe the tumors would have shrunk. We will never know. We were deprived of the opportunity to find out.

Cancer Inhibitors

Agrimony

Rapid bone repair in a patient with lung cancer metastases to the spine using a novel herbal medicine: A case report. Oncol Lett. 2016 Sep ;12(3):2023-2027. Epub 2016 Jul 18. PMID: 27602132

Astragalus

Effect of astragalus injection combined with chemotherapy on quality of life in patients with advanced non-small cell lung cancer. Zhongguo Zhong Xi Yi Jie He Za Zhi. 2003 Oct;23(10):733-5. PMID: 14626183

Baicalein

Baicalein increases cisplatin sensitivity of A549 lung adenocarcinoma cells via PI3K/Akt/NF-κB pathway. Biomed Pharmacother. 2017 Jun ;90:677-685. Epub 2017 Apr 14. PMID: 28415048

Bamboo

Aqueous extract of Bambusae Caulis in Taeniam (bamboo shavings) inhibits PMA-induced tumor cell invasion and pulmonary metastasis: suppression of NF-κB activation through ROS signaling. PLoS One. 2013 ;8(10):e78061. Epub 2013 Oct 28. PMID: 24205091

Bee Venom

Melittin exerts an antitumor effect on non-small cell lung cancer cells. Mol Med Rep. 2017 Sep ;16(3):3581-3586. Epub 2017 Jul 14. PMID: 28713976

Melittin suppresses tumor progression by regulating tumor-associated macrophages in a Lewis lung carcinoma mouse model. Oncotarget. 2017 Jun 27. Epub 2017 Jun 27. PMID: 28666252

Berberine

Effect of berberine on activity and mRNA expression of N-acetyltransferase in human lung cancer cell line A549. J Tradit Chin Med. 2014 Jun ;34(3):302-8. PMID: 24992757

Breathing Exercises

Morning breathing exercises prolong lifespan by improving hyperventilation in people living with respiratory cancer. Medicine (Baltimore). 2017 Jan ;96(2):e5838. PMID: 28079815

Carotenoids

Inverse Association between Dietary Intake of Selected Carotenoids and Vitamin C and Risk of Lung Cancer. Front Oncol. 2017 ;7:23. Epub 2017 Feb 28. PMID: 28293540

Afterward Notes

Cherry

Effect of acerola cherry extract on cell proliferation and activation of ras signal pathway at the promotion stage of lung tumorigenesis in mice. J Nutr Sci Vitaminol (Tokyo). 2002 Feb;48(1):69-72. PMID: 12026193

Chinese Medicine

Integrated Chinese-western therapy versus western therapy alone on survival rate in patients with non-small-cell lung cancer at middle-late stage. J Tradit Chin Med. 2013 Aug ;33(4):433-8. PMID: 24187861

Cruciferous Vegetables

Cruciferous vegetable intake is inversely associated with lung cancer risk among smokers: a case-control study. BMC Cancer. 2010 ;10:162. Epub 2010 Apr 27. PMID: 20423504

Cruciferous Vegetable Intake Is Inversely Associated with Lung Cancer Risk among Current Nonsmoking Men in the Japan Public Health Center Study. J Nutr. 2017 Apr 5. Epub 2017 Apr 5. PMID: 28381528

Pre-diagnostic cruciferous vegetables intake and lung cancer survival among Chinese women. Sci Rep. 2015 ;5:10306. Epub 2015 May 19. PMID: 25988580

Cucurbitacin

Cucurbitacin B regulates immature myeloid cell differentiation and enhances antitumor immunity in patients with lung cancer. Cancer Biother Radiopharm. 2012 Oct ;27(8):495-503. Epub 2012 Jun 29. PMID: 22746287

Fruits and Vegetables

Intakes of fruits, vegetables, and related vitamins and lung cancer risk: results from the Shanghai Men's Health Study (2002-2009). Nutr Cancer. 2013 ;65(1):51-61. PMID: 23368913

Risk of lung cancer and consumption of vegetables and fruit in Japanese: a pooled analysis of cohort studies in Japan. Cancer Sci. 2015 May 29. Epub 2015 May 29. PMID: 26033436

Garlic

Raw garlic consumption and lung cancer in a Chinese population. Cancer Epidemiol Biomarkers Prev. 2016 Jan 25. Epub 2016 Jan 25. PMID: 26809277

Ginger

6-shogaol, an active constituent of dietary ginger, impairs cancer development and lung metastasis by inhibiting the secretion of CC-chemokine ligand 2 (CCL2) in tumor-associated dendritic cells. J Agric Food Chem. 2015 Feb 18 ;63(6):1730-8. Epub 2015 Feb 9. PMID: 25621970

Isoflavones

Isoflavone intake and risk of lung cancer: a prospective cohort study in Japan. Am J Clin Nutr. 2010 Jan 13. Epub 2010 Jan 13. PMID: 20071645

Moringa

A potential oral anticancer drug candidate, Moringa oleifera leaf extract, induces the apoptosis of human hepatocellular carcinoma cells. Oncol Lett. 2015 Sep ;10(3):1597-1604. Epub 2015 Jul 10. PMID: 26622717

Melatonin

HDAC1 inhibition by melatonin leads to suppression of lung adenocarcinoma cells via induction of oxidative stress and activation of apoptotic pathways. J Pineal Res. 2015 Jul 16. Epub 2015 Jul 16. PMID: 26184924

Mushroom

The use of mushroom glucans and proteoglycans in cancer treatment. Altern Med Rev. 2000 Feb;5(1):4-27. PMID: 10696116

Sporoderm-Broken Spores of Ganoderma lucidum (Reishi mushroom) Inhibit the Growth of Lung Cancer: Involvement of the Akt/mTOR Signaling Pathway. Nutr Cancer. 2016 Oct ;68(7):1151-60. Epub 2016 Aug 11. PMID: 27618151

Anticancer activity of Amauroderma rude (mushrooms). PLoS One. 2013 ;8(6):e66504. Epub 2013 Jun 20. PMID: 23840494

Inhibitory effect of a water-soluble extract from the culture medium of Ganoderma lucidum mycelia (Reishi mushroom) on the development of pulmonary adenocarcinoma induced by N-nitrosobis (2-hydroxypropyl) amine in Wistar rats. Oncol Rep. 2006 Dec;16(6):1181-7. PMID: 17089035

Piperine

Piperine induces apoptosis of lung cancer A549 cells via p53-dependent mitochondrial signaling pathway. Tumour Biol.

2014 Apr ;35(4):3305-10. Epub 2013 Nov 24. PMID: 24272201

Resveratrol (red grape skins among others)

Resveratrol in lung cancer- a systematic review. J BUON. 2016 Jul-Aug;21(4):950-953. PMID: 27685918

4'-Chloro-3,5-dihydroxystilbene, a resveratrol derivative, induces lung cancer cell death. Acta Pharmacol Sin. 2010 Jan;31(1):81-92. PMID: 20048747

Shikonin

Clinical trial on the effects of shikonin mixture on later stage lung cancer. Zhong Xi Yi Jie He Za Zhi. 1991 Oct ;11(10):598-9, 580. PMID: 1806305

Soy

Soy intake is associated with lower lung cancer risk: results from a meta-analysis of epidemiologic studies. Am J Clin Nutr. 2011 Dec ;94(6):1575-83. Epub 2011 Nov 9. PMID: 22071712

Soy consumption and mortality in Hong Kong: proxy-reported case-control study of all older adult deaths in 1998. Prev Med. 2006 Jul;43(1):20-6. Epub 2006 May 2. PMID: 16631248

Soy consumption reduces the risk of non-small-cell lung cancers with epidermal growth factor receptor mutations among Japanese. Cancer Sci. 2008 Jun;99(6):1202-8. Epub 2008 Apr 21. PMID: 18429954

Tea

Afterward Notes

Tea consumption and lung cancer risk: a meta-analysis of case-control and cohort studies. Nutrition. 2014 Oct ;30(10):1122-7. Epub 2014 Mar 12. PMID: 25194612

Vitamin B

Serum B vitamin levels and risk of lung cancer. JAMA. 2010 Jun 16 ;303(23):2377-85. PMID: 20551408

Vitamin C

Association between vitamin C intake and lung cancer: a dose-response meta-analysis. Sci Rep. 2014 ;4:6161. Epub 2014 Aug 22. PMID: 25145261

Restoring physiological levels of ascorbate slows tumor growth and moderates HIF-1 pathway activity in Gulo(-/-) mice. Cancer Med. 2015 Feb ;4(2):303-14. Epub 2014 Oct 30. PMID: 25354695

Vitamin D

Vitamin d and lung cancer risk: a comprehensive review and meta-analysis. Cell Physiol Biochem. 2015 ;36(1):299-305. Epub 2015 May 4. PMID: 25967968

Ecological Studies of the UVB-Vitamin D-Cancer Hypothesis. Anticancer Res. 2012 Jan ;32(1):223-36. PMID: 22213311

Vitamin E

Dietary vitamin E intake could reduce the risk of lung cancer: evidence from a meta-analysis. Int J Clin Exp Med. 2015 ;8(4):6631-7. Epub 2015 Apr 15. PMID: 26131295

Cancer Promoters

High Fat Diet

High-fat Diet Enhances and Plasminogen Activator Inhibitor-1 Deficiency Attenuates Bone Loss in Mice with Lewis Lung Carcinoma. Anticancer Res. 2015 Jul ;35(7):3839-47. PMID: 26124329

Lactose Intolerance (in other words avoiding dairy decreases risk, implying dairy may promote cancer)

Lactose intolerance and risk of lung, breast and ovarian cancers: aetiological clues from a population-based study in Sweden. Br J Cancer. 2014 Oct 14. Epub 2014 Oct 14. PMID: 25314053

Low Cholesterol (do cholesterol lowering drugs promote cancer?)

Low plasma cholesterol predicts an increased risk of lung cancer in elderly women. Prev Med. 1995 Nov ;24(6):557-62. PMID: 8610078

Pesticides

Occupational Exposure to Pesticides and the Incidence of Lung Cancer in the Agricultural Health Study. Environ Health Perspect. 2016 Jul 6. Epub 2016 Jul 6. PMID: 27384818

Radiotherapy

Ionizing radiation and tobacco use increases the risk of a subsequent lung carcinoma in women with breast cancer:

case-only design. J Clin Oncol. 2005 Oct 20;23(30):7467-74. PMID: 16234513

Statins

Exposure to statins and risk of common cancers: a series of nested case-control studies. BMC Cancer. 2011 ;11:409. Epub 2011 Sep 26. PMID: 21943022

Sugar

Increased sugar uptake promotes oncogenesis via EPAC/RAP1 and O-GlcNAc pathways. Yasuhito Onodera, Jin-Min Nam and Mina J. Bissell. J Clin Invest. 2014 Jan 2; 124(1): 367–384. Published online 2013 Dec 9. doi: 10.1172/JCI63146. PMCID: PMC3871217. PMID: 24316969

A9 Practical Lessons

> You were always the one who stood back and helped when I needed help, ... any little (or big) thing I needed.
>
> ~ Beverly Kaiman

Disclaimer: I am not a doctor, lawyer, accountant, financial adviser, or other certified professional. This is not professional advice. You should consult with the appropriate professionals.

My lifelong friend Steven Wurgler suggested including some notes on lessons learned.

When you are facing this situation for the first time, you do not know what to do. Part of the appeal is that Hospice is going to take care of everything for you. You can just go home. Hospice will bring over everything you need.

You do not need to panic. You do not need to jump into Hospice's comforting arms right away. You can take your time to consider your options. You can find assistive equipment online, fairly inexpensively. You can get home healthcare independently. You can have your own doctor.

See the doctors that know the most about your condition. Get multiple opinions. If someone tells you they cannot help you, look for someone else.

Get tests done. Find out what is going on. There are tests that can detect cancer cells in your blood stream long before tumors can be detected on a scan. There are people that will test your cancer against chemotherapy drugs and natural substances to find out which ones work on your cancer cells in a petri dish.

Afterward Notes

If your patient is immobile, get an automatically inflating air mattress to prevent bed sores. Trying to prevent bed sores yourself is too difficult.

In brief:

Cancer is not an immediate death sentence

1. Do not accept other people's hopelessness

2. Do not give up

3. Life is a death sentence

4. Live your life to the end

5. Not every pain is cancer, most are not

6. You may be able to slow, or even reverse, your tumor growth

Get your papers in order early

1. Medical power of attorney

2. Financial power of attorney

3. Living will to pull the plug

4. Regular will to distribute assets

5. Beneficiaries on investment accounts

6. Survivors' names on bank accounts

7. Bill of sale for the car

8. Bill of sale for household and personal items

9. In states that allow have a deed upon death for the house

Make up your mind to preserve relationships

1. You are going to disagree on things that are important to you

2. Argue, fight, you will win some and lose some

3. Respect who has the authority to make which decisions

4. Do not hold grudges, let the past go

Eat Healthy

1. Food is medicine

2. Eat whole foods: Create a healthy body environment that is inhospitable to cancer

3. Organic fruits, vegetables, nuts, seeds, legumes, beans, whole grains, herbs, fermented foods

4. Some cancer fighting foods are cruciferous vegetables, broccoli, cauliflower, Brussels sprouts, leafy greens, kale, spinach, flax seeds, ginger, turmeric with black pepper, garlic, onions, leeks, beets, carrots, sweet potatoes, lemon, berries, cranberries, pomegranate, hibiscus, green tea, moringa

Afterward Notes

Avoid toxic foods

1. Refined carbohydrates, refined sugar

2. Added salt and chemicals

3. Fried foods, added fats

4. Meats especially burned, farmed fish, chicken

5. Dairy and eggs not from organic, free-range animals

6. Processed foods

7. Produce that is not organic due to the pesticides, depleted soils

Eat questionable foods only occasionally, weekly or less

1. Fish would be good but is polluted

2. Meat, dairy, eggs from organic, free range animals with natural diets

Get a nutritional profile and address deficiencies

1. Omega 3 fats are low in our diets

2. Vitamin B and B12 in particular are low on vegan diets

3. Vitamin C is low because we do not eat enough fruit

4. Vitamin D is low because we do not get enough sun

Avoid unnecessary drugs

1. Avoid addiction

Avoid Toxins

1. Avoid blue light at night

2. Avoid plastic containers

3. Avoid toxic chemicals in your house, on your lawn, in your pool

4. Check what you are putting on your skin

5. Test your air

6. Test your home for Radon

7. Test your water

Exercise

1. Get your heart rate up, both moderate and high intensity

2. Stretch

3. Sweat

4. Walk

5. Weight Lift

Afterward Notes

Go Outside

1. Breath fresh air

2. Get in the sun for 15 minutes each day with exposed skin

3. Swim in the ocean, lakes, rivers, springs

4. Walk in the woods

Holistic and Alternative Treatments

1. Create a healthy environment physically and emotionally

2. Acupuncture

3. Aroma therapy

4. Essential oils

5. Hypnosis

6. Light

7. Massage

8. Music

9. Non-mainstream therapies

Research online

1. Beware

2. Check research studies

3. Find alternative cancer research

4. Find nutrition experts

5. Find people in similar situation

6. Find support groups

Sleep

1. Dark, quiet

2. Dream

Socialize

1. Go to your church, synagogue or wherever

2. Live your life

3. Use support groups

4. Visit with family and friends

A10 Palliative Care Verses Hospice Care

The following explanation is taken from the National Cancer Institute website as is on September 12, 2016. There is no copyright notice on the page. Since the information is on a government website, I believe the information to be in the public domain. This notice appears on the page "Most text on the National Cancer Institute website may be reproduced or reused freely. The National Cancer Institute should be credited as the source."

From the NIH - National Cancer Institute

http://www.cancer.gov/about-cancer/advanced-cancer/care-choices/palliative-care-fact-sheet

Palliative Care in Cancer

- What is palliative care?

- When is palliative care used in cancer care?

- Who gives palliative care?

- If a person accepts palliative care, does it mean he or she won't get cancer treatment?

- What is the difference between palliative care and hospice?

- Where do cancer patients receive palliative care?

- How does a person find a place that offers palliative care?

- What issues are addressed in palliative care?

- Can a family member receive palliative care?

- How is palliative care given at the end of life?

- How do people talk about palliative care or decide what they need?

- Who pays for palliative care?

- Is there any research that shows palliative care is beneficial?

What is palliative care?

Palliative care is care given to improve the quality of life of patients who have a serious or life-threatening disease, such as cancer. The goal of palliative care is to prevent or treat, as early as possible, the symptoms and side effects of the disease and its treatment, in addition to the related psychological, social, and spiritual problems. The goal is not to cure. Palliative care is also called comfort care, supportive care, and symptom management.

When is palliative care used in cancer care?

Palliative care is given throughout a patient's experience with cancer. It should begin at diagnosis and continue through treatment, follow-up care, and the end of life.

Who gives palliative care?

Afterward Notes

Although any medical professional may provide palliative care by addressing the side effects and emotional issues of cancer, some have a particular focus on this type of care. A palliative care specialist is a health professional who specializes in treating the symptoms, side effects, and emotional problems experienced by patients. The goal is to maintain the best possible quality of life.

Often, palliative care specialists work as part of a multidisciplinary team to coordinate care. This palliative care team may consist of doctors, nurses, registered dieticians, pharmacists, and social workers. Many teams include psychologists or a hospital chaplain as well. Palliative care specialists may also make recommendations to primary care physicians about the management of pain and other symptoms. People do not give up their primary care physician to receive palliative care.

If a person accepts palliative care, does it mean he or she won't get cancer treatment?

No. Palliative care is given in addition to cancer treatment. However, when a patient reaches a point at which treatment to destroy the cancer is no longer warranted, palliative care becomes the total focus of care. It will continue to be given to alleviate the symptoms and emotional issues of cancer. Palliative care providers can help ease the transition to end-of-life care.

What is the difference between palliative care and hospice?

Although hospice care has the same principles of comfort and support, palliative care is offered earlier in the disease process. As noted above, a person's cancer treatment continues to be administered and assessed while he or she is receiving palliative care. Hospice care is a form of palliative care that is given to a person when cancer therapies are no longer controlling the disease. It focuses on caring, not curing. When a person has a terminal diagnosis (usually defined as having a life expectancy of 6 months or less) and is approaching the end of life, he or she might be eligible to receive hospice care. More information is available in the National Cancer Institute (NCI) fact sheet Hospice Care.

Where do cancer patients receive palliative care?

Cancer centers and hospitals often have palliative care specialists on staff. They may also have a palliative care team that monitors and attends to patient and family needs. Cancer centers may also have programs or clinics that address specific palliative care issues, such as lymphedema, pain management, sexual functioning, or psychosocial issues.

A patient may also receive palliative care at home, either under a physician's care or through hospice, or at a facility that offers long-term care.

How does a person find a place that offers palliative care?

Patients should ask their doctor for the names of palliative care and symptom management specialists in the community. A local hospice may be able to offer referrals as well. Area hospitals or medical centers can also provide information. In addition, some national organizations have specific databases for referrals. For example, the Center to Advance Palliative Care has a list of providers by state.

What issues are addressed in palliative care?

Palliative care can address a broad range of issues, integrating an individual's specific needs into care. The physical and emotional effects of cancer and its treatment may be very different from person to person. For example, differences in age, cultural background, or support systems may result in very different palliative care needs.

Comprehensive palliative care will take the following issues into account for each patient:

Physical. Common physical symptoms include pain, fatigue, loss of appetite, nausea, vomiting, shortness of breath, and insomnia. Many of these can be relieved with medicines or by using other methods, such as nutrition therapy, physical therapy, or deep breathing techniques. Also, chemotherapy, radiation therapy, or surgery may be used to shrink tumors that are causing pain and other problems.

Emotional and coping. Palliative care specialists can provide resources to help patients and families deal with the emotions that come with a cancer diagnosis and cancer treatment. Depression, anxiety, and fear are only a few of the concerns that can be addressed through palliative care. Experts may provide counseling, recommend support groups, hold family meetings, or make referrals to mental health professionals.

Practical. Cancer patients may have financial and legal worries, insurance questions, employment concerns, and concerns about completing advance directives. For many patients and families, the technical language and specific details of laws and forms are hard to understand. To ease the burden, the palliative care team may assist in coordinating the appropriate services. For example, the team may direct patients and families to resources that can help with financial counseling, understanding medical forms or legal advice, or identifying local and national resources, such as transportation or housing agencies.

Spiritual. With a cancer diagnosis, patients and families often look more deeply for meaning in their lives. Some find the disease brings them more faith, whereas others question their faith as they struggle to understand why cancer happened to them. An expert in palliative care can help people explore their beliefs and values so that they can find a sense of peace or reach a point of acceptance that is appropriate for their situation.

Can a family member receive palliative care?

Yes. Family members are an important part of cancer care, and, like the patient, they have a number of changing needs. It is common for family members to become overwhelmed by the extra responsibilities placed upon them. Many find it difficult to care for a relative who is ill while trying to handle other obligations, such as work and caring for other family members. Other issues can add to the stress, including uncertainty about how to help their loved one with medical situations, inadequate social support, and emotions such as worry and fear. These challenges can compromise their own health. Palliative care can help families and friends cope with these issues and give them the support they need.

How is palliative care given at the end of life?

Making the transition from curative treatment to end-of-life care is a key part of palliative care. A palliative care team can help patients and their loved ones prepare for physical changes that may occur near the end of life and address appropriate symptom management for this stage of care. The team can also help patients cope with the different thoughts and emotional issues that arise, such as worries about leaving loved ones behind, reflections about their legacy and relationships, or reaching closure with their life. In addition, palliative care can support family members and loved ones emotionally and with issues such as when to withdraw cancer therapy, grief counseling, and transition to hospice. For more information, see the NCI PDQ® information summary Last Days of Life.

How do people talk about palliative care or decide what they need?

Patients and their loved ones should ask their doctor about palliative care. In addition to discussing their needs for symptom relief and emotional support, patients and their families should consider the amount of communication they need. What people want to know about their diagnosis and care varies with each person. It is important for patients to tell their doctor about what they want to know, how much information they want, and when they want to receive it.

Who pays for palliative care?

Palliative care services are usually covered by health insurance. Medicare and Medicaid also pay for palliative care, depending on the situation. If patients do not have health insurance or are unsure about their coverage, they should check with a social worker or their hospital's financial counselor.

Is there any research that shows palliative care is beneficial?

Yes. Research shows that palliative care and its many components are beneficial to patient and family health and well-being. A number of studies in recent years have shown that patients who have their symptoms controlled and are able to communicate their emotional needs have a better experience with their medical care. Their quality of life and physical symptoms improve.

In addition, the Institute of Medicine 2007 report Cancer Care for the Whole Patient cites many studies that show patients are less able to adhere to their treatment and manage their illness and health when physical and emotional problems are present.

A11 Robert Dentmond 911 Call

911 Call Made by Robert Dentmond Before He Was Killed By Police

https://www.youtube.com/watch?v=LfEaIYxZkLM

Posted by YouTube member TentyOne

Published on May 2, 2016

552 views as of October 30, 2016

This is the recording of the 911 call 16-year-old Robert Dentmond placed to the Alachua County Sheriff's Office on March 20, 2016. During the call, he tells the dispatcher he's suicidal and had an M-16 rifle. He was shot and killed by 4 police officers a short time later.

Police press release:

"At approximately 10:07 PM last evening, the Alachua County Sheriff's Office Combined Communications Center (CCC) received a 9-1-1 call from Robert Dentmond who stated to call takers that he was walking around the Majestic Oaks Apartment Complex with an "M-16" rifle. Mr. Dentmond also advised CCC personnel that he wanted to shoot himself then disconnected the line.

Several ACSO patrol units were dispatched to the scene. Shortly after arrival, an ACSO patrol supervisor encountered Mr. Dentmond who was armed with what appeared to be an AR-15 style assault rifle. Several additional patrol units from both the Alachua County Sheriff's Office and the Gainesville

Police Department responded as backup. Deputies and Officers began a dialogue with Mr. Dentmond who initially dropped his weapon after verbal commands were issued. Responding units attempted to establish a rapport with Mr. Dentmond to get him to step away from the weapon. After several minutes of dialogue, Mr. Dentmond picked up the weapon, arming himself, and began to walk toward one of the occupied apartment buildings inside the complex. Deputies and Officers with both agencies proceeded to again give a series of loud verbal commands directing Mr. Dentmond to drop the weapon. Mr. Dentmond did not respond to the directions he was given and began to, again, walk toward an occupied apartment building within the complex.

Mr. Dentmond was given several warnings by Deputies and Officers that they were not going to let him approach an occupied apartment complex while armed. Mr. Dentmond was given multiple opportunities to stop, accompanied by several warnings that Deputies and Officers would be forced to fire if he continued towards the occupied building while armed. Deputies and Officers made it extremely clear to Mr. Dentmond that if he continued to walk towards the occupied apartment building carrying the rifle, they would have no other option but to utilize deadly force. As a result of Mr. Dentmond's refusal to comply with the directions of Deputies and Officers, lethal force was utilized to stop the threat Mr. Dentmond posed to residents of the complex. Deputies and Officers immediately rendered medical aid to Mr. Dentmond who was treated and transported by Alachua County Fire Rescue to UF Health at Shands Hospital where he was later pronounced deceased.

Afterward Notes

The investigation into the officer involved shooting has been turned over to the Florida Department of Law Enforcement. The ACSO Office of Professional Standards and GPD's Internal Affairs will also conduct an administrative investigation into the incident pending the conclusion of FDLE's investigation. As a matter of routine procedure, ACSO Deputies and GPD Officers involved in the lethal use of force will be placed on temporary administrative duties within their respective departments until such time as the investigations are concluded."

A12 Donations in Memory of Edith Weitzen

Marjorie Bars and Phil Kabler - Youth Fund

Ruth Berman and Connie Kurtz - Dora Geld Friedman Religious School, Congregation B'nai Israel

Nancy and Gabriel Bitton - Aesthetics Fund, Congregation B'nai Israel

Carol Bleichfeld - Rabbi's Discretionary Fund, Congregation B'nai Israel

Tatiana Borisova - Congregation B'nai Israel

Libby Brateman - Friendship Circle Fund, Congregation B'nai Israel

Patti and Fred Brownstein - Rabbi's Discretionary Fund, Congregation B'nai Israel

Suzanne Chester - Dora Geld Friedman Religious School, Congregation B'nai Israel

Gail and Harvey Cohen - The Pap Corps, Champions of Cancer Research, UM Sylvester Cancer Center, Bellaggio Chapter

Jerry and Sherry Cohen - Social Action Fund, Congregation B'nai Israel

Marian and Howard Cohen- Kiddish Fund, Congregation B'nai Israel

Afterward Notes

Congregation B'nai Israel Sisterhood - Torah Fund Campaign of Women's League for Conservative Judaism

Stan and Jodi Cullen - Cemetery Beautification Fund, Congregation B'nai Israel

Cindy and Jordan Dern - Kiddish Fund, Congregation B'nai Israel

Lori and Mike Dribin - Rabbi's Discretionary Fund, Congregation B'nai Israel

Morris Sternberger, Marvin Goldstein, Alan Sternberger and Drew, Sharon, Joshua and Shaina Fein - Jewish National Fund, Trees for Israel

Freda Green - Rabbi's Discretionary Fund, Congregation B'nai Israel

Hadassah Gainesville Chapter - Hadassah

Ann and Marc Heft - Rabbi's Discretionary Fund, Congregation B'nai Israel

Leslie and Dee Dee Hendeles - Youth Fund, Congregation B'nai Israel

Jill Hirsh - Kiddish Fund, Congregation B'nai Israel

Rebecca and Richard Howard - Kiddush Fund, Congregation B'nai Israel

Gilda Josephson - Cemetery Beautification Fund, Congregation B'nai Israel

Beverly and Marvin Kaiman - Ed Chester Library Fund, Congregation B'nai Israel

Elaine Kaplan - Congregation B'nai Israel Programming, Congregation B'nai Israel

Ruth Kovacs - Jewish National Fund, Trees for Israel

Dawn Burgess-Krop and Harry Krop - Pew Plaque in the Congregation B'nai Israel Sanctuary

Nicole and Maurice Levy - Congregation B'nai Israel Programming Fund, Congregation B'nai Israel

Roslyn and Norman Levy - Cemetery Beautification Fund, Congregation B'nai Israel

Phyllis Lotzkar - Cemetery Beautification Fund

Valerie Messina - Congregation B'nai Israel Programming Fund, Congregation B'nai Israel

Richard and Dorothy Melker - Rabbi's Discretionary Fund, Congregation B'nai Israel

Alan and Debra Mibab - Jewish National Fund, Trees for Israel

Nancy and Kevin Milner - Cemetery Beautification Fund, Congregation B'nai Israel

Scott and Anne-Beth Nemerhoff - B'nai Israel Programming Fund, Congregation B'nai Israel

Arnost and Susan Neugroschel - Rabbi's Discretionary Fund, Congregation B'nai Israel

Afterward Notes

Barbara Oberlander - Kiddish Fund, Congregation B'nai Israel

Beth Oettinger and Family - Jewish National Fund, Trees for Israel

Laura Preisler - Na'amat USA

Judy and Bill Page - Rabbi's Discretionary Fund, Congregation B'nai Israel

David and Harriett Pawliger - Ed Chester Library Fund, Congregation B'nai Israel

Linda Ramsy - Keren Kayemeth LeIsrael (JNF), Trees for Israel

Jaquie and Michael Resnick - Torah Fund Campaign of Women's League for Conservative Judaism

Nadine and Des Schatz - B'nai Israel Programming Fund, Congregation B'nai Israel

Eleanor R Schmidt - Cemetery Beautification Fund, Congregation B'nai Israel

Mark and Ruth Sherwood - Rabbi's Discretionary Fund, Congregation B'nai Israel

Sandy and John Shuster - Cemetery Beautification Fund, Congregation B'nai Israel

Carol and David Silverman - Kiddish Fund, Congregation B'nai Israel

Phil and Roz Slater - B'nai Israel Sisterhood, Congregation B'nai Israel

Marvin Slott - Rabbi's Discretionary Fund, Marvin Slott

Eric and Lynne Sobel - Kiddish Fund, Congregation B'nai Israel

Connie and Bob Stern - Community Day School, Congregation B'nai Israel

Jill and Scott Tomar - Two Shabbat Siddurs, Congregation B'nai Israel

Phyllis and Mickey Warren - Dora Geld Friedman Religious School, Congregation B'nai Israel

Kenneth Wald and Robin West - Kiddish Fund, Congregation B'nai Israel

Michael and Elaine Zimmerman - Botanical Garden of Palm Beach County

My apologies to anyone left off this list. Let me know so I can update.

A13 Issues

In this book I have provided eyewitness evidence, in which Hospice serves as a proxy for bad behavior prevalent in the medical industry. My complaint is not with mistakes, which can happen to anyone, but with method, which is systemic. Issues come in many forms such as failure to put the patient as an individual first, misrepresentation, lack of accountability, lack of oversight, insistence of knowledge that is not there, failure to acknowledge they do not know what they are doing with medications, treating of symptoms instead of causes, training doctors to memorize but not think, ignorance of health, and ignorance of nutrition.

Issues with the Hospital

From Chapter 4 Too Late

1. Over medication as a matter of practice when under medication should be the norm.

Issues with the Doctor

From Chapter 5 Smoke and Mirrors

1. Making an unqualified diagnosis of how long Mom was going to live based on criteria for acceptance to Hospice's care.

Issues with Hospice

Chapter 5 Smoke and Mirrors

1. Not putting the patient's interest first.

2. Misrepresenting what they do.

3. Misrepresenting what is going to happen to you under their care.

4. Depriving my mother of making an informed decision.

Chapter 6 Oncologists

1. Depriving my mother of seeing the oncologist.

Chapter 7 Oxycodone

1. Giving my mother Oxycodone.

2. Irresponsibly prescribing drugs.

3. Prescribing medication without seeing the patient.

4. Not having holistic treatment for pain management.

5. Not having respect for the patient as an individual.

Chapter 8 Radiation Therapy

1. Over medicating my mother.

2. Turning my mother into a drug addict.

3. Depriving my mother of a chance to face her situation.

4. Depriving my mother of living her life after successful radiation therapy.

Afterward Notes

Chapter 9 Drug Addiction

1. Not acknowledging their incompetence in misreading my mother's medical reports.

2. Their assuredness in pronouncing how long my mother had to live.

3. Treating patients for the convenience of the caretakers.

4. Going about business as usual, ignoring my mother's drug addiction when I raised the issue.

5. Stealing my mother's mind.

6. Depriving us of a chance to save my mother.

Chapter 10 Hospice Staff

1. Not listening to the patient.

2. Their determination in sticking to their agenda.

Chapter 11 Family and Friends

1. Depriving my mother's friends of seeing my mother.

2. Depriving us, her family, of spending meaningful time with her.

3. Depriving my mother of spending meaningful time with family and friends.

Chapter 12 Keep Comfortable

1. Shutting down my mother's digestive system.

2. Keeping my mother bedridden.

3. Causing my mother to lose all her muscle.

4. Causing my mother unnecessary pain.

Chapter 14 Nutrition

1. Their lack of respect for nutrition.

Chapter 15 Lorazepam

1. Giving my mother Lorazepam.

Chapter 16 Doctor Death

1. Their arrogance.

2. Not heeding warnings.

3. Putting my mother back on drugs once she was off them.

4. Depriving us of a chance to save my mother.

5. Repeating the same errors.

6. Giving my mother worse drugs.

Chapter 17 Alprazolam

1. Giving my mother Alprazolam.

2. Ignorantly prescribing a drug without calculating dosage amounts.

3. Addicting my mother to yet another drug Alprazolam.

Chapter 18 Methadone

1. Giving my mother Methadone.

2. Not giving my mother a chance to get better.

3. Taking away my mother's mind a second time.

4. Shutting down my mother's digestive system intentionally.

5. Inducing my mother's tumors to grow faster.

6. Causing my mother to develop severe bed sores.

7. The misery they put my mother through.

8. Poisoning my mother with opioids.

9. Making my mother die from lack of water.

10. Killing my mother, who I believe would be alive as I write this.